BODY COMPOSITION IN SPORT, EXERCISE AND HEALTH

The analysis of body composition (fat, bone and muscle) is an important process throughout the biomedical sciences. This is the first book to offer a clear and detailed introduction to the key methods and techniques in body composition analysis and to explain the importance of body composition data in the context of sport, exercise and health.

With contributions from some of the world's leading body composition specialists, the book goes further than any other in demonstrating the practical and applied value of body composition analysis in areas such as performance sport and weight control in clinical populations. The book pays particular attention to the important concept of change in body composition, and includes discussion of ethical issues in the collection, interpretation and presentation of data, and considerations when working with special populations.

Bridging the gap between research methods and practical application, this book is important reading for advanced students and practitioners working in sport and exercise science, health science, anatomy, nutrition, physical therapy and ergonomics.

Arthur D. Stewart has worked in body composition as an editor of the *Journal of Sports Sciences*, for the International Olympic Committee's working group on body composition, and as criterion anthropometrist and Vice President of the International Society for the Advancement of Kinanthropometry. He has over 60 publications, including his recent research in 3D body scanning at Robert Gordon University, UK.

Laura Sutton completed her PhD in body composition analysis, in the process working with a wide variety of populations including recreational and elite athletes, disability groups, the fire service and the armed forces. Laura currently works as a medical statistician at the University of Liverpool, UK.

BODY COMPOSITION IN SPORT, EXERCISE AND HEALTH

*Edited by Arthur D. Stewart and
Laura Sutton*

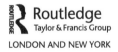

Routledge
Taylor & Francis Group

LONDON AND NEW YORK

First published 2012
by Routledge
2 Park Square, Milton Park, Abingdon, Oxon OX14 4RN

Simultaneously published in the USA and Canada
by Routledge
711 Third Avenue, New York, NY 10017

Routledge is an imprint of the Taylor & Francis Group, an informa business

British Library Cataloguing in Publication Data
A catalogue record for this book is available from the British Library

Library of Congress Cataloging in Publication Data
A catalog record has been requested for this book

ISBN: 978-0-415-61497-9 (hbk)
ISBN: 978-0-415-61498-6 (pbk)
ISBN: 978-0-203-13304-0 (ebk)

Typeset in Bembo
by Saxon Graphics Ltd, Derby

DEDICATION

We wish to dedicate this book to the memory of Professor Tom Reilly, Liverpool John Moores University. You have been an inspiration to us, and so many others within academia. We thank you for cultivating our interest in body composition, for your diligence, your professionalism, your humour and being the unsung mentor without whom neither of us could have entertained this project. This book was your idea, and we hope that in taking on this venture, some of your enthusiasm can reach its wider readership.

CONTENTS

FIGURES AND TABLES

Figures

Tables

NOTES ON CONTRIBUTORS

J.E. Lindsay Carter
School of Exercise and Nutritional Sciences San Diego State University, USA.
Chapter 4: Physique: phenotype, somatotype and 3D scanning.

Vicky L. Goosey-Tolfrey
The Peter Harrison Centre for Disability Sport, Sir John Beckwith Centre for Sport, School of Sport Exercise and Health Sciences, Loughborough University, UK.
Chapter 9: Body composition in chronic disease and disability.

Patria A. Hume
Sport Performance Research Institute New Zealand, School of Sport and Recreation, Faculty of Health and Environmental Sciences, AUT University, New Zealand.
Chapter 8: Body composition change.

Mike Marfell-Jones
Open Polytechnic, Kuratini Tuwhera, New Zealand.
Chapter 7: Anthropometric surrogates for fatness and health.

Yvonne Mulholland
Centre for Obesity Research and Epidemiology, Robert Gordon University, UK.
Chapter 3: Portable methods of body composition analysis.

Alan M. Nevill
University of Wolverhampton, School of Sport, Performing Arts and Leisure, UK.
Chapter 7: Anthropometric surrogates for fatness and health.

Catherine Rolland
Centre for Obesity Research and Epidemiology, Robert Gordon University, UK.
Chapter 2: Laboratory methods of body composition analysis; Chapter 3: Portable methods of body composition analysis.

Arthur D. Stewart
Centre for Obesity Research and Epidemiology, Robert Gordon University, UK.
Chapter 1: The concept of body composition and its applications; Chapter 4: Physique: phenotype, somatotype and 3D scanning; Chapter 7: Anthropometric surrogates for fatness and health; Chapter 8: Body composition change; Chapter 10: Body composition: professional practice and an interdisciplinary toolkit.

Laura Sutton
Department of Biostatistics, Institute of Translational Medicine, Faculty of Health & Life Sciences, University of Liverpool, UK.
Chapter 5: Muscle tissue; Chapter 6: Bone tissue; Chapter 9: Body composition in chronic disease and disability; Chapter 10: Body composition: professional practice and an interdisciplinary toolkit.

FOREWORD

It is a privilege and pleasure to write the foreword for this book on Body Composition in Sport, Exercise and Health. It is poignantly dedicated to the memory of the great Professor Tom Reilly, who generated the idea and original outline for the book, shortly before he died in 2009. Thanks to the editors Dr Arthur Stewart and Dr Laura Sutton, the project has been continued to successful completion and this book now sits among one Tom's many valuable initiatives and contributions to sport and exercise science. Among many of his other successful interests in sports science, Tom was most interested in kinanthropometry and the validity of methods of assessing body composition. As everyone who knew him would attest, he was also profoundly interested in the academic and professional development of his students and his colleagues. It is therefore so fitting and such apt testimony to Tom Reilly's legacy of mentoring staff and students, that this should continue by bringing together one of his many recent PhD graduates (Laura Sutton) with his colleague Arthur Stewart, an established practitioner and researcher in body composition and 'criterion' anthropometrist with the International Society for the Advancement of Kinanthropometry. Arthur and Laura have assembled a team, which includes some leading specialists in the field, to produce an informative source of reference for students and practitioners from a range of professions. The content spans descriptions of a range of the most practicable techniques for assessing body composition and physique, considered within the context of how these factors are changed through health and exercise and within special populations. Editors Arthur Stewart and Laura Sutton and their contributors are to be warmly congratulated on a worthy contribution to this field of interest. Well done to you! Tom Reilly would be most proud of you and the outcome you have produced.

Professor Roger Eston
Sansom Institute for Health Research,
School of Health Sciences,
University of South Australia,
Adelaide

PREFACE

The application of science to the different realms of health and performance has dramatically pushed back the frontiers in both domains. What we are made of in terms of our constituents and their relative proportions has a profound influence over our health and our capability for exercise. The science of body composition is seldom viewed as such, yet has a unique bridge-building role to link practitioners from a wide variety of disciplines. It is this diversity which renders our subject so rich and exciting, yet which makes writing a volume dedicated to it so challenging. While some texts either embrace a single measurement approach, and others go into the considerable detail of physics of each measurement technique, this book seeks to strike a balance that presents the science in a useful summary, and is practitioner-focused.

This book systematically deals with definitions and frames of context (Chapter 1) before summarising the key measurement techniques for laboratory based and field based assessment of body composition (Chapters 2 and 3). Somatotype and phenotype are combined in a single chapter, which traces the development of this area and includes the relevance of 3D scanning for current and future research. Muscle and bone tissue are considered in discrete chapters, and in addition to describing how these compartments are measured, they include detail of anatomy, physiology and the relationship with growth and performance. Chapter 7 considers what many might view as the most vocationally-relevant section – on surrogates for adipose tissue (including the ISAK 2011 protocol for skinfolds), detailing how adiposity might be assessed without recourse to calculating a percentage fat, which inevitably includes a range of assumptions, some of which might not be justified. Chapter 8 considers the change in body composition associated with growth, ageing and performance, and introduces a framework for explaining the dynamic nature of physique and body composition. Chapter 9 is an area all-too-readily overlooked in science – the specifics of the measurements of disabled individuals for body composition and considerations for effective measurement. Chapter 10 has a focus on the professional practice that relates to body composition assessment, and includes a range of approaches and exemplars which will assist professionals in their work.

We hope that with the balanced contents above, this book will be an effective reference for practitioners across a range of professions, including physiology, biomechanics, nutrition and dietetics, strength and conditioning, and others. With professional organisation input, this book can be rightfully considered as a guide, equally suited to researcher or practitioner.

ACKNOWLEDGEMENTS

We wish to record our thanks to all our chapter contributors who share our collective interest in body composition, and without whom writing this book would have been infinitely more difficult. We gratefully acknowledge Robert Gordon University and the University of Liverpool for their support in enabling us to complete the project. We would also like to thank the International Society for the Advancement of Kinanthropometry and the British Association of Sport and Exercise Sciences for permission to use their input. Thanks go to our colleagues and participants whose co-operation has been essential in developing our practical and academic skills in body composition. Finally, we would like to thank Taylor and Francis, specifically Joshua Wells and Simon Whitmore, for their initiative, expertise and encouragement throughout the publication process.

ABBREVIATIONS

3DPS	three-dimensional photonic scanning
^{3}H	tritium
ADNFS	Allied Dunbar national fitness survey
ADP	air displacement plethysmography
AFFST	appendicular fat-free soft tissue
AIDS	acquired immune deficiency syndrome
ASIA	American Spinal Injury Association
ATP	adenosine triphosphate
BASES	British Association of Sport and Exercise Sciences
BIA	bioelectric impedance analysis
BIS	bioimpedance spectroscopy
BMC	bone mineral content
BMD	bone mineral density
BMI	body mass index
BMR	basal metabolic rate
C	carbon
Ca	calcium
CAT	computed axial tomography
CF	cystic fibrosis
CI	conicity index
Cl	chlorine
CO_2	carbon dioxide
COPD	chronic obstructive pulmonary disease
COSHH	control of substances hazardous to health
CT	computed tomography
CVD	cardiovascular disease
D_2O	deuterium

DOMS	delayed onset muscle soreness
DPA	dual-photon absorptiometry
DXA	dual X-ray absorptiometry
ECW	extracellular water
FFM	fat-free mass
FFMI	fat-free mass index
FFST	fat-free soft tissue
FM	fat mass
H	hydrogen
HIV	human immunodeficiency virus
HSE	Health and Safety Executive
HWR	height-weight ratio
IAF	intra-abdominal fat
ICW	intracellular water
ISAK	International Society for the Advancement of Kinanthropometry
ISBCR	International Society for Body Composition Research
ISCD	International Society for Clinical Densitometry
IVNA	in vivo neutron activation
KeV	Kilo-electronvolts
kHz	kilohertz
LREC	local research ethics committee
MHC	myosin heavy chain
MHz	megahertz
MeV	Mega-electronvolts
MF	multi-frequency
MRI	magnetic resonance imaging
ms	milliseconds
N	nitrogen
Na	sodium
NHS	National Health Service
NIR	near infrared interactance
nm	nanometre
NRES	National Research Ethics Service
O	oxygen
P	phosphorus
QALY	quality-adjusted life year
QCT	quantitative computed tomography
QDR	quantitative digital radiography
QUS	quantitative ultrasound
RF	radio frequency
RPI	reciprocal ponderal index
SAA	surface area artefact
SAD	somatotype attitudinal distance (Chapter 4)
SAD	sagittal abdominal diameter

SAM	somatotype attitudinal mean
SAT	subcutaneous adipose tissue
SCI	spinal cord injury
SEE	standard error of the estimate
SF	single frequency
SXA	single X-ray absorptiometry
TBK	total body potassium
TBW	total body water
TE	total error
TEE	total energy expenditure
TEM	technical error of measurement
TOBEC	total-body electrical conductance
UWW	underwater weighing
VAT	visceral adipose tissue
WC	waist circumference
WHO	World Health Organization
WHR	waist-to-hip ratio
WSR	waist-to-stature ratio

1

THE CONCEPT OF BODY COMPOSITION AND ITS APPLICATIONS

Arthur D. Stewart

This chapter will cover:

1.1   Introduction
1.2   History of body composition research
1.3   Influences on human physique
1.4   Definitions and approaches
1.5   Applications of body composition

1.1 Introduction

Why body composition?

To some, body composition might seem an obscure branch of anatomy or physiology, less exciting than other branches of science which are in the public consciousness. However, a close look at body composition reveals not a dry, static science, but a vibrant, dynamic area, of research which targets the entire spectrum of scale from the atom to the population. It is a science with a rich history and great practical relevance today, and its analytical processes cut to the very heart of some fundamental, philosophical and controversial issues.

- Should the occupational health test have a threshold of fatness above which employees are not able to work in certain environments?
- At what level of fatness does childhood obesity become an issue of child protection?
- How should the International Olympic Committee approach the issue of changes to competition rules, because of unhealthy practices in athletes achieving competition weight?

• Why are black athletes superior to white athletes at track sprinting, but white athletes superior to black athletes at swimming?

As we consider these questions, it becomes clear that the answers are not straightforward. Throughout this book, we will explore the science which provides the evidence which will enable us to address these questions. However, we need to recognise that it is not necessarily the scientist who has to answer them. Only in the last question will science provide a possible answer, while in the first three, judgements regarding implementing change have to be made bearing in mind other factors such as legal obligation, precedent and consequences. In clinical practice, a dichotomous decision is required in any test for the presence or absence of a disease. In the case of obesity, we can arrive at the simple yes/no answer by applying a test designed to predict those who are obese. However, in any sample there are likely to be those who have the disease and test negative (false negatives) and those who do not have the disease and test positive (false positives), the relative numbers of which affect how the test is used. For the scientist in practice, dichotomous decisions are rare, and more common is the need to quantify a parameter or factor affecting health or performance across a spectrum of data values. The different perspectives of the clinician and scientist are important in answering the three controversial questions above, but any model which culminates in a dichotomous decision needs to be based on robust science which is reproducible and valid, as well as being open to scrutiny. Such a model will need to quantify the parameters in question, and identify common principles, as well as the effect size and scope for individual variability.

While this might appear sound, a further layer of complexity is introduced when we consider that the human body does not remain fixed in terms of body composition. Rather, it exhibits changes with growth, ageing, exercise, energy balance, etc. which are implicit in the definition of the health of any living organism (see Section 1.4). It also alters as a consequence of forces exerted on it – most noticeably when the 1-2 per cent diurnal variation in stature is observed as a consequence of gravitational forces progressively compressing structures in the spine when upright (Tyrrell, Reilly & Troup, 1985). Gravity also influences the fluid components of the body and less rigid tissues, such that posture can influence body composition measurements. Carin-Levy et al. (2008) demonstrated such a difference in standing and supine skinfold measures, which is an important consideration in certain patient groups such as stroke victims. The issue of how to assess body composition in disabled groups is discussed in more detail in Chapter 9.

Now we can begin to appreciate that measuring the human body is not as straightforward as it sounds, both because of the need to standardise the influences on the body at the time of measurement, such as fasting and hydration status, and also the approaches to the measurements themselves. The topics addressed in this book seek not only to describe the approaches and limitations used in a range of methods, but provide detail on the real-life questions that quantifying body tissues can inform. The importance and sensitivity of such questions addressed by the science of body composition today have never been greater. The implication of scientific findings of body composition, both in health and in sport have never been so far-reaching.

1.2 History of body composition research

Since Hippocrates attributed health to an appropriate balance of four body fluids, the study of the constituent parts of the body has fascinated scientists and medics. While medicine has undergone relentless progress, and Hippocrates' ideas might seem strange by contemporary understanding, it is a measure of his remarkable insight to consider how many of the issues that he observed relating to diet and exercise in particular, still hold true today.

Throughout the history of civilisation, we see some evidence of human obesity – but it was so rare that it was revered as god-like, and almost certainly confined to political leaders and royalty. For instance, the Venus of Willendorf is an 11 cm high statuette of an obese female figure estimated to have been crafted at least 22,000 years ago. Discovered in 1908 by archaeologist Joseph Szombathy at a Paleolithic site near Willendorf, Austria, it was carved from limestone not found in the local area, and subsequently tinted with red ochre. Whatever value might have been attributed to this artifact, it is likely that such a select individual as depicted would have enjoyed a position of political influence, affording the luxury of feasting as a matter of routine, while being spared the physical outlay demanded of the majority. For most early civilisations, however, the imperatives for deriving food and water prevailed, alongside a large energy expenditure necessary to fulfil the needs of migration or military combat.

As civilisation became more developed, farming became more efficient, enabling the prospect of cultural elaboration. In ancient Greece, fascination with the body form and the concept of physical perfection resulted in intricate statues being produced in a systematic way. Polykleitos (460–410 BC) created a new approach to sculpture encapsulated in a treatise (or canon) to exemplify his aesthetic theory of the mathematical bases of perfection. This contended that a statue should comprise clearly definable parts, all related to one another through a system of ideal mathematical proportions and balance. His best known work *Doryphorus*, the spear bearer, with an ideal physique (based on several individuals, exemplifying the canon) 'suitable for war and athletics' symbolises the early origins of anthropometric measurement. However, the contribution of the Ancient Greek civilisation was to be much greater than that of aesthetics and art. Archimedes (c.287–212 BC) correctly observed that the buoyant force on a submerged object equals the weight of the water it displaces, enabling the calculation of its specific gravity. He thus pioneered the science of densitometry, correctly observing that King Hiero's crown was in fact an alloy which included cheaper and less dense metals and was not pure gold. The same science would be developed for use with the whole body in the mid-twentieth century. In the Renaissance period, Leon Battista Alberti (1404–1471) created the *Definer*, which comprised a skull cap and protractor with an extendable rule with and plumb lines. This enabled radial and vertical distance to be accurately plotted to key landmarks. As a result, statues could be mathematically 'encoded' and replicated to different sizes in different locations.

The first systematic body composition study was in 1921, when Jindrich Matiegka developed a validated method of quantifying bone, muscle and adipose tissue, together with residual mass (Matiegka, 1921). He used the classical anatomical approach (see Section 1.4) and he applied this to quantify tissue variability in barbers, blacksmiths, hairdressers and gymnastics instructors. However, his imperative was to examine the efficiency of the body in terms of work production, which was important in order to assess human capability in times of military conflict in the aftermath of the First World War.

Albert Behnke (1924–1992) was a military physician with the US Navy whose interests and achievements were mostly in the field of hyperbaric medicine. As part of this, he discovered the elimination of inert gas was affected by fat content and physical fitness. His achievements included developing a hydrostatic method for assessing fatness based on Archimedes' principle, as well as a metric for composition of healthy college-age males and females, derived from large scale military and civilian surveys data, referred to as *reference man* and *reference woman* (Behnke and Wilmore, 1974). This quantified the constituents in a typical male and female, and such an approach was not to create an ideal value, so much as a yardstick against which individuals could be compared. His contribution to the field means that he is considered by many to be the 'modern day father of body composition'.

Josef Brozek (1913–2004) was a researcher in fields of nutrition and psychology. He undertook a range of psychological studies during the Minnesota starvation study of the mid-1940s which sought to induce semi-starvation and study rehabilitation strategies against a background of chronic food shortage after the Second World War. In parallel with other work to model fat mass by William Siri, he developed a formula for relating measured density to fatness. Both conversions are still in use today and the method is discussed in detail in Chapter 3.

Alongside the major efforts to compartmentalise the body's constituents, the body's phenotype and physique were investigated by a number of individuals, relating shape to discrete patterns of body types, which generally recognised slenderness, muscularity and fatness separately. Although these had long been observed, they were related to personality by Ernst Kretschmer (1888–1964) and involved a gradation between normality and psychoses. Popularisation of the term 'somatotype' is credited to William Sheldon (1898–1977) who contended that a person's physique was predestined. He developed a physique classification system based on nude photographs of the body in standard poses. Controversy over the procedure, and the use of the photographs (his subjects were mostly Ivy League students) led to the Smithsonian Institute subsequently destroying the collection. Physique classifications were later developed using anthropometry by Barbara Heath (1919–1998) and J.E. Lindsay Carter, as discussed in Chapter 4.

During the 1970 and 1980s, the densitometric method was developed for body-fat prediction purposes, and large studies involving skinfolds which were used to predict fat content as measured by underwater weighing were developed in the UK by Durnin & Womersley (1974) and the USA by Jackson & Pollock (1978) and Jackson, Pollock & Ward (1980). At this time, densitometry was viewed as a valid criterion method against which other methods could legitimately be compared. However since this time, the adequacy of the two-compartment method and several of the assumptions upon which it is based have been called into question, as detailed in Chapter 2.

In the 1980s, a further dimension to our understanding was added with the advent of the Brussels Cadaver Study. This involved a total of 25 male and female cadavers undergoing full anatomical dissection, with the separate compartments weighed and analysed. The magnitude of this work, because of the nature of dissection work, and the care and exactitude required, is rarely appreciated. The fact that multiple anthropometric measurements were made on the cadavers which enabled the estimation of muscle, bone as well as adipose tissue, skin and fat, enabled a raft of subsequent publications to produce mass fractionation predictions on the skinfold (Clarys, Martin, Drinkwater & Marfell-Jones, 1987), muscle mass (Martin, Spenst, Drinkwater & Clarys, 1990), and the skeletal mass (Drinkwater & Ross, 1986).

Appreciating that the cadaver dissection represents the absolute against which all methods should be compared, the Brussels Cadaver Study remains the largest and most robust investigation to use this method. However, the challenges of predicting body composition in living humans, especially healthy or athletic adults or children, meant that its relevance was called into question for many avenues of research. Against this backdrop, the development of dual X-ray absorptiometry (DXA) emerged at the start of the 1990s, with the capability for total and regional *in vivo* composition. This three-compartment method was to be compared against densitometry, and bore the aspirations of many researchers in the field of body composition for becoming the reference method of choice. Although cadavers have been analysed using DXA, its main validation was against the carcasses of pigs which were subsequently chemically analysed. This enabled direct measurement of bone mineral and fat, while the remaining fat-free soft tissue could predict muscle mass with reasonable accuracy. While DXA remains a popular method today, its limitations (discussed in Chapter 2) are not always fully appreciated.

When the total body mass is fractionated into components, there is a balance to be struck between the number of components which can be assessed in living humans, and the added value to a meaningful composition calculation. Most researchers would probably agree that a four-compartment model (water, fat, bone mineral and fat-free soft tissue) is adequate for most applications, although requirements may be mandated by circumstances. For instance, in radiological protection work, occupational health screening requires the detection of individual elements. The methods used for multi-component models are considered in Chapter 2.

1.3 Influences on human physique

In biological systems there is a relationship between the numbers within a species and the available food supply. Wild animals are faced with the pressure to compete for the food, to migrate to alternative supply locations and avoid predation. This places the food supply and consumption environment in a delicate balance, which is collectively influenced by a range of factors within the ecosystem. However, if an animal were to become domesticated, this balance would alter, and the genetic programming governing eating behaviour would not be accompanied by the need to migrate or defend food supply. Humankind, sharing over 98 per cent of the genetic code of the lower primates, is no different. Our remarkable biology has enabled us to thrive on exercise and an intermittent food supply, preserving sufficient stored fat to enable migration to a new geographical region where food might be abundant, without impeding the capacity for exercise itself. Today, by contrast, we can appreciate the limiting nature of those suffering morbid obesity, who find basic ambulatory locomotion a major challenge and may have effectively surpassed the 'tipping point' of being too heavy to be capable of using exercise to assist in energy balance. The obesity pandemic in the Western world is testimony to such redundant biology, which perfectly prepares us for famine that never arrives.

As humankind developed social structures and technologies for agriculture, transportation, warfare and medicine, the driving imperatives for our biological mechanisms became less influential in terms of body composition and physique. Today, although physical performance may be less influential in military conflict than weapon technology, the requirement for infantry troops to be capable of demanding physical outlay requiring strength, endurance and agility is still paramount. Paradoxically, while the vast majority of Western populations remain sedentary and at risk of becoming overweight or obese, there has been a commensurate proliferation of seemingly incredible physical achievements, either in ultra-endurance sport, expeditions or survival. These have helped define our understanding of the limits of what is humanly possible, how trainable are key parameters, from health, occupational or sports performance perspectives.

The intricate construction of the human body, which has served the species so well during its evolutionary history, enables physique to be a dynamic phenomenon, adapting to variability in food availability and energy expenditure via their consequent effects on metabolism. In anthropology, the detailed study of indigenous species has uncovered a wealth of knowledge about such adaptation – in terms of morphology which is largely genetic (such as stature and proportionality of the skeletal system), or environmental (such as muscle and adipose tissue accumulation). Beyond the rigidity or plasticity of such tissues, the physiological load imposed by environmental temperature, pressure and even altitude are forces which have been considered to shape human physique.

Although it is widely believed that stature is genetically determined, in contemporary Western societies, approximately 20 per cent of the variability in stature can be attributable to the environment (Silventoinen, 2003). Historic census data from the mid-nineteenth century collected before the American Civil War explored brothers' height in relation to county population (Lauderdale and Rathouz, 1999). Using data from 3,898 Union soldiers, including 595 with multiple brothers, they found stature decreased with county population size (P < 0.001) and that the correlation between brothers' heights decreased significantly with increasing county population, while the variance increased. Likely mechanisms could include limited energy supply or increased energy expenditure, and the environmental contribution to variability in height was noted to be more influential in poorer environments. Around the same time, the German zoologist Christian Bergmann (1814–1856) identified a link between body size of mammals and birds and latitude. 'Bergmann's rule' was best explained by the surface area to volume ratio, which affects heat exchange, and would favour smaller mammals at lower latitudes. Exceptions to the rule were considered to have other compensatory mechanisms operating – which include behavioural adaptations. Nevertheless, such assertions have remained controversial, and within the human species consideration of the low stature of the Inuit of Northern Canada and high stature of various African tribal peoples, suggests such an analysis may be overly simplistic. Observed indigenous groups display complex variation, although such ethnic distinctions have become less apparent in the last 50 years or so with the increasing mixing of the gene pool.

Over a similar period of time, a commensurate alteration in occupational activity for much of the world population has resulted from the mechanisation of work, while introduction of labour-saving devices, motorised transport, central heating and other adaptations, have all served to reduce individual energy expenditure. On the other side of the energy balance equation, advances in food manufacture and processing, combined with persuasive marketing of highly palatable energy-dense food, have occurred, resulting in the increasing prevalence and progression of obesity. If hundreds of thousands of years of evolution have crafted our species to thrive on an oscillating pattern of exercise and rest, coupled with an intermittent food supply, where migration to a new food source was implicit, today's uncoupling of food acquisition and exercise has de-emphasised a range of regulatory mechanisms, and must be seen as something of an evolutionary own goal for *Homo sapiens*. The chronic overweight, over-fat phenotype with centralised abdominal obesity, with multiple health risks has caused some to propose the evolution of a new species *Homo adipatus* is underway (Broom & Rolland, 2010). These researchers represent current thinking in metabolic research which recognises adipose tissue as an endocrine organ, manufacturing signalling molecules which control energy metabolism, immune function and reproduction. Accumulation of excessive fat produces a pro-inflammatory state which interferes with such mechanisms at a cellular level and is destructive to health.

While the effects of the obese phenotype are obvious enough, a musculo-skeletal system which has not been forced to adapt to the exercise stimuli is not only weaker, it has to withstand the greatly increased energy cost and work requirements of carrying a heavier body. Although it is widely recognised that obese individuals do far less physical activity than those of a normal weight, researchers have debated which is the cause and which is the effect. Does obesity cause inactivity, or does inactivity cause obesity? Although the answer is not always clear, there is persuasive evidence for both. The effects of inactivity have been shown to overwhelm those of physical activity participation, because individuals tend to be sedentary for much longer than they are active. An interview-based study of 3,392 adults from the Australian state of New South Wales found associations between body mass index (BMI) and physical activity with hours of TV watched. Respondents in the low, moderate and high physical activity categories who reported watching more than four hours or television per day were twice as likely to be overweight, compared to those who watched less than one hour, irrespective of physical activity participation (Salmon, Bauman, Crawford, Timpiero & Owen, 2000, pp. 600, 604).

1.4 Definitions and approaches

Body composition is considered by some to mean 'level of fatness' but it is important to consider the other components too. Its more appropriate and full definition is much wider than this: 'the chemical or physical components that collectively make up an organism's mass, defined in a systematic way' (Stewart, 2010, p. 455). Its utility is therefore 'a metric for categorising the body into meaningful sub-units' which is likely to include either lipid or adipose tissue alongside others. The extensive medical, physiological, and nutritional literature using different body composition methods has provided great insight as to the relationship between body constituents in health and disease, but because the body can be subdivided using different approaches, it is an essential first step to understand whichever one is used in a given study or data set.

Anatomical approach. This is the classical approach performed by a series of great anatomists over the last few centuries, largely within the context of universities' medical schools. This considers the different tissue masses as they could be dissected from a fresh cadaver, enabling separate identification of skin, adipose tissue, muscle, bone and residual tissue masses.

Chemical approach. This approach assumes no method in particular but divides the body into a number of subcategories of similar chemicals. The starting point for both is the whole body, but whereas the anatomical approach yields four, five or six components at most, the chemical approach can ultimately yield every chemical element within the body.

Compartmental models are created from different approaches, whereby the body is subdivided as far as appropriate for the task, and the cost involved. For most purposes, there might be a requirement for two, three or four categories. For instance for a sports scientist, it might be important to consider variation in muscularity, skeletal proportions and fatness, while for a clinician with haemodialysis patients, total body water, intracellular and extracellular water are more appropriate.

In some circumstances, a single elemental content is required – for instance to assess safe levels of exposure to heavy metals.

What it is important to establish, before any detail of methods of assessing body composition is outlined, is the hierarchy between the whole body and the chemical elements which represent the smallest reducible unit. This concept is referred to as the *level of analysis*, and was conceived by Wang, Pierson & Heymsfield (1992). Several variations on this model exist, one of which is illustrated in Figure 1.1.

Whole body and body regions. The body can be treated as an entity on its own or alternatively it can be subdivided into discrete anatomical regions. In densitometry the body is treated as a whole for the calculation of whole-body density. By contrast, the approach commonly taken for medical students studying anatomy considers discrete regions, where the interrelationships of all tissues and constituents are considered. This is fundamental in clinical contexts, for example the consideration of injury, where a spinal injury at a certain level may affect specific muscles, nerves and reflexes which have consequences for normal functioning. In terms of the gross anatomy, a dual X-ray absorptiometry (DXA) scan enables subdivisions of the scan so different regions can be considered separately. However two limitations of this need to be appreciated. First, the precision of where the cut-lines are placed depends upon the pixel size of the instrument – and these are generally ~1 cm across, so differences between contra-lateral arms may be merely a

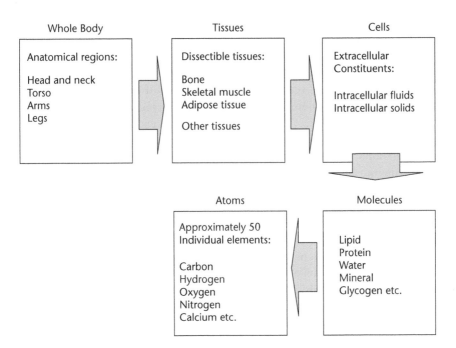

Whole Body	Tissues	Cells
Anatomical regions: Head and neck Torso Arms Legs	Dissectible tissues: Bone Skeletal muscle Adipose tissue Other tissues	Extracellular Constituents: Intracellular fluids Intracellular solids

Atoms	Molecules
Approximately 50 Individual elements: Carbon Hydrogen Oxygen Nitrogen Calcium etc.	Lipid Protein Water Mineral Glycogen etc.

FIGURE 1.1 An example of the levels of analysis approach whereby the whole body is divided into its constituents.

function of this limitation, and the lines between torso and arms may not be in equivalent locations. Second, the junction between body segments is not normally in a perpendicular plane, so any vertical division of the orthogonal scan, will include some torso tissue in arms and vice versa.

Tissues and organs represent the first sub-level of organisation. Muscle tissue is normally the most abundant tissue in the body, commonly accounting for between a third and a half of total body mass. Adipose tissue and skeletal tissue, in addition to muscle, comprise approximately three-quarters of mass in most healthy individuals, with the remaining mass representing internal organs. However, such proportions may alter dramatically in the extremes of body composition – in the case of chronic undernourishment, muscle tissue is metabolised to fulfil energy requirement, and in extreme examples of morbid obesity, adipose tissue itself can represent three-quarters of body mass.

Muscle tissue comprises several thousand individual contractile muscle fibres, bound together within a sheath of connective tissue. Skeletal or striated muscles are arranged in bundles of fibres, each of which contains hundreds of thread-like protein strands called myofibrils. When an impulse from a motor nerve reaches the muscle, action potentials are generated which cause contraction. Muscles have the capacity to generate much more force than is commonly observed, and have a synchronised stimulus–relaxation pattern which serves to protect against injury and fatigue.

Adipose tissue is a form of connective tissue comprising adipocytes, arranged in lobules. It is located beneath the skin in the subcutaneous depot, and deeper than the peritoneum, around the internal organs in the visceral depot. The visceral depot represents discrete developmental layers which may be referred to separately. These include the omental fat associated with the greater and lesser omenta – which are layers of peritoneum which pass from the stomach and the first part of the duodenum to the other viscera, arranged in an apron around the stomach, or the intra- and retro-peritoneal fat, within or posterior to the peritoneum, respectively. Adipose tissue has a blood supply, and both elastin and collagen fibres to provide shape. Plasticity of adipose tissue is important in facilitating movement, and the sheathing fasciae of adjacent tissues also serve to anchor adipose tissue and constrain movement. The lipid fraction of adipocytes varies with cell size, and is different within and between individuals. As a consequence, this affects tissue density and several of the available measures for assessing adiposity. If skinfolds are considered as worthy surrogates for fatness, then further considerations are necessary as regards skin thickness. While in most individuals, the subcutaneous depot is much larger, accumulation in the visceral depot represents a much greater health risk (Björntorp, 1997). It is a common misconception that adipose tissue is equivalent to fat, but this is not the case. Several key differences were explored in a study of 34 cadavers and 40 comparable-aged living volunteers, which highlighted that compressibility and fat content of skinfolds were variable, and skin thickness greater in men than women (Clarys, Provyn & Marfell Jones, 2005).

Skeletal tissue is another form of connective tissue, which has several functions including providing support, protection and the storage of mineral. Bone combines the strength of mineral (calcium hydroxyapatite) with the flexibility of collagen to create a material which is stronger than hard wood or concrete, and is one third of the weight of cast iron (Einhorn, 1996). Bone tissue is arranged in two distinct architectures: *trabecular* bone, which comprises interconnecting cross plates (trabeculae) and the solid *cortical* bone, which are explained in more detail in Chapter 6. These varieties facilitate different functions of metabolically active bone, and the less active role required for protection. Optimising the skeletal structure is an imperative for all vertebrates and involves a compromise between strength and the energetic cost of movement.

Cells represent what is often considered to be the autonomous functional unit of the body. Survival of any multicellular organism requires different cells to assume different functions. In complex organisms, such specialisation determines the anatomy of the cell, as well as how its activity responds to signals from its environment. While it is beyond the scope of this chapter to consider the cell differentiation pathways, it is noteworthy that in humans, cell types are fundamentally different in morphology. Adipocytes are fat cells containing the lipid store, the individual muscle myofibrils are muscle cells, and living bone has three major types of cells, osteoblasts, osteoclasts and osteocytes. While Chapters 5 and 6 will include more detail on these, most applications of body composition techniques do not require cellular mass to be quantified. However, for various approaches, quantification of extra and intracellular fluid is important – for instance in haemodialysis patients.

Molecules exist in the body in over 100,000 varieties, however the principal five are, in decreasing order of abundance, water, protein, lipid, mineral and carbohydrate. Although lipid is mainly triglyceride, other essential lipids include phospholipids and cholesterol which have different chemical structures and greater density. Lipids are defined as molecules which do not dissolve in water, but are soluble in organic solvents such as ether.

Elements exist in variable abundance in the human body. Although there are approximately 50 in total, 98 per cent of body mass is comprised of only six, namely hydrogen, carbon, oxygen, nitrogen, phosphorous and calcium (Eston, Hawes, Martin & Reilly, 2009). This approach is used to quantify protein by its nitrogen content, and this together with a range of other elements including carbon, sodium, phosphorous, chlorine and calcium can be assessed by neutron activation analysis. This involves bombarding the participant with neutrons which induce the release of radio-isotopes which can be measured during or after the neutron irradiation. By contrast, potassium 40 radiation occurs naturally and can be measured as it exits the body. Facilities for elemental analysis are rare, and their use restricted to specialist composition measurements, for example screening for contamination by Cobalt 60 for nuclear industry or defence workers involved in decommissioning reactors.

As well as these units for considering body composition data, we must also focus on a range of definitions which apply to scientific measurements, including accuracy, precision, reliability and validity.

Accuracy represents the actual or true value. It is quantified by comparing a reference method with a prediction method. It is also important to appreciate that the true measurement may change over time.

Precision represents the error associated with repeated measurements and is quantified as the observed variability of repeated measures made on the same person. It has the same as units of measurement e.g. millimetres or coefficient of variation (standard deviation/mean), expressed as a percentage. Low variability means high precision and vice versa.

Reliability is similar to precision, but is usually presented as a correlation coefficient (especially the 'intraclass' correlation coefficient) which has no units, and whose values also depend on the variability of measures within the subject group being measured.

Validity is the extent to which a measurement is representative of a particular characteristic or quantity for which the true value is known.

One of the main challenges in the field of body composition is that different analytical methods measure properties at different levels within this hierarchy before arriving at a body composition measurement. While this might at first appear as though a simple conversion is needed, when we consider a definition of health (see Section 1.5), we see that the concentrations of one unit of measurement – for example the potassium content of fat-free mass, or the lipid content of adipose tissue - can vary by at least 15 per cent. As a consequence of such variation, methods cannot legitimately be equated nor converted between levels without assumptions, which presume that the variation has been constrained and quantified. For instance, anthropometric skinfolds of superficial adipose tissue are linear distances. Densitometry involves measuring whole body density, and relating this to percentage fat by assuming the density of all tissues excluding fat is constant. DXA involves measuring the attenuation of X-rays which operate at the molecular level which enables discriminating bone mineral (calcium hydroxyapatite) and lipid from other molecules (both approaches are described in Chapter 2). A study which develops a prediction of densitometry or DXA-derived fat from skinfolds or bioimpedance must therefore take cognisance of the assumptions and error of both the predictor method (skinfolds) and the dependent variable (DXA or densitometry), and not merely assume that the latter is accurate. This reality is not always appreciated in body composition research, and particularly in applications of clinical or sporting practice which are farther from the laboratory setting. In truth, the tools of the trade of the body composition scientist are neither as precise nor as accurate as we would wish, and some are indeed 'blunt' instruments when applied at the individual level. The misinformation resulting from data which are poorly interpreted, or the presumption of accuracy of reference methods are issues which continue to threaten our understanding and professional practice.

1.5 Applications of body composition

The paradigms of health and sport are different, and this distinction is important when it comes to the application of knowledge or body composition data.

Health, as defined in *Blakiston's Pocket Medical Dictionary* is:

'the state of dynamic equilibrium between an organism and its environment which maintains its structural and functional integrity between certain end limits'

(Igoe, 1979, p. 358)

Optimising health is a difficult concept to quantify. On the other hand, the absence of health or risk factors for disease can be quantified in terms of morbidity or mortality. Morbidity, or disability can be quantified in functional tests of, for example strength, eyesight etc. and impact calculated in the relative risk of acquiring disease, or quality-adjusted life year (QALY). Mortality can be quantified in terms of age at death, or the odds ratio of premature death. For instance, we know that for calculating the likelihood of certain diseases, epidemiologists will frequently use a BMI scale (X axis) to describe population risk (Y axis). This might enable a comparison of relative risk between groups, against BMI, for example in smoking as in the theoretical example illustrated in Figure 1.2.

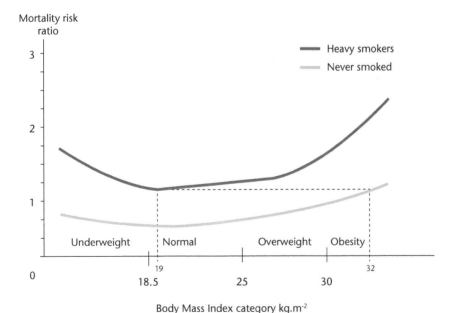

FIGURE 1.2 Mortality risk in heavy smokers versus those who have never smoked, compared by body mass index.

In this illustration, a non-smoker has a similar mortality risk as a smoker with a BMI of 13 fewer units – which means for the same mortality risk as the lowest of a smoker, a non-smoker would be 35 kg heavier. However, the full picture is not that simple, because there is an interaction between BMI and smoking, especially at higher levels of BMI.

By comparison, sports performance is more easily defined. Optimising sports performance generally uses either outcome data, for example winning or making a final, or performance criteria, such as time, distance or weight, although in aesthetic sports, appearance, poise and other factors are of concern. In biomechanical terms, athletes are attempting to achieve one or more of a small number of challenges. These include achieving maximum strength, maximum power, maximum velocity, minimum energy expenditure etc. In order to comply with such biomechanical imperatives, athletes and coaches are usually very aware of the power: weight ratio, and optimising the body mass and composition for the requirements of the task. Underpinning the perfect sports performance is the perfect physique, which optimises the size, and minimises excess fat in order to fulfil these biomechanical imperatives. As a consequence of this, sport may be demanding the body to comply with drivers that might run counter to those supporting health. This relationship is described in terms of percentage body fat in Figure 1.3.

This disparity was illustrated by George Sheehan MD (1918–1993) who famously said, "Runners who look well are at least five pounds overweight, and on their way to being happy and contented and psychologically invulnerable. I want no part of that." He alludes to an important point relating sports performance to a gaunt and possibly undernourished appearance. As we will discover in Chapter 8, optimising the physique for performance is unsustainable in terms of long-term health, in the same way as a mountaineer cannot stay on the summit of a Himalayan peak indefinitely, but must return to lower altitudes in order to recover from the environmental stresses exerted.

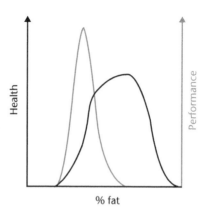

FIGURE 1.3 The relation of percentage fat to health and performance.

Health

In a wider health arena, modelling body composition at the population level can provide important information regarding increased disease risk which may have consequences for morbidity, mortality and health care costs. The use of indices for assessing adiposity is addressed in Chapter 7, by illustrating the point, we could consider the effect of an increase in BMI as it affects disease risk. While it is widely understood that morbid obesity carries an additional health risk, such analysis can enable understanding of how modest increases within a nominally healthy BMI range can precipitate disease. What is also interesting is to note that disease risk affects different ethnic groups differently, because of the inherent limitations of the body mass index (which does not measure composition, only relative mass). Asians would appear to experience health risks at lower BMI possibly as a result of greater genetic susceptibility and also a slender frame reducing their BMI for a given level of fatness.

Ergonomics is the science concerned with optimising the human–machine interface in a health-sustaining way. As health in the workplace is becoming an increasingly important issue for employers as well as employees, there is an increased emphasis on all aspects of health at work. Different work environments demand different considerations, in terms of workstation configuration in computing and location, orientation, visibility of controls and warning information for industrial machines, together with the strength and dexterity required to perform physical tasks. Transportation policymakers require to be informed of population trends in body size, weight and, by implication, composition. The Civil Aviation Authority considers the *seat pitch* – the distance between one aircraft passenger seat and the same position on the adjacent row, with respect to emergency egress. Consideration of the loading of winches in ships' lifeboats needs to anticipate the total mass of a full complement of passengers. Both these examples are considered on a probability basis, where the likelihood of having an atypical size spectrum of people is calculated. It is noteworthy that newer designs of hospital beds and wheelchairs are larger and better able to support more obese patients. However, in the built environment too, it is important to recognise that within the lifespan of machines (for example lifts), the population has become taller (values of about 8 mm per decade in many Westernised countries have been reported, but such trends do not usually remain constant) and substantially heavier as a consequence. The safety margin built into the lift design for load carrying will become substantially reduced during the lifetime of the lift, and in most countries is routinely inspected and certified for use. Thankfully incidents which are attributable to load failure are extremely rare, due to the effective legislation concerned. However, in various other industrial settings, including circumstances routinely faced by the emergency services, strenuous work in confined spaces mean compromised safety for those attending any incident. Evacuating larger and heavier casualties is more challenging, more time consuming, and increases risk exposure to all concerned.

Exercise and sport: the fit-fat distribution

It is widely recognised that exercise plays a vital role in developing and maintaining fitness, and that this is protective against injury or disease risk. It is also well understood that exercise helps maintain a 'positive' body composition, by maintaining the integrity of bones, maintaining muscle mass and helping to maintain energy balance, without which the progression to excess body fat is more apparent. However, as well as exercise influencing fat quantity, it can also have an effect on its distribution. Nindl and colleagues (1996) measured body composition on elite infantry recruits who were required to undergo a regime of prolonged intense physical training and energy deficit dietary intake. What they discovered was the hierarchy of use of the different regional fat depots on the body – beginning with the abdomen, followed by the arms and lastly the legs. This pattern had already been recognised in an earlier study of Norwegian recruits (Rognum, Rodahl & Opstad, 1982), but Nindl's group compared the distribution between elite troops and less-fit regular infantry soldiers with the same overall level of fatness. The elite recruits had less abdominal fat and greater arm fat, relative to less-fit individuals. This confirmed not only the order of recruitment of fat from regional depots, but the presence of the 'fit-fat distribution' as a phenomenon which appeared to be in equilibrium, without a prevailing energy deficit. Taken together, these findings have implications for predicting adiposity across samples of variable fitness, as well as recognising serious threats to health in terms of undernourishment by identifying depletion of regional depots – which can be done using field-based techniques in developing countries. Although there is no implication of local recruitment of fat depots by active musculature beyond isolated deposits of intramuscular fat, these findings, combined with biochemical evidence of greater lipolytic activity in abdominal fat confirm that exercise appears to diminish the effect of the potentially harmful abdominal deposition of fat. This underscores the need to predict fatness from active and sedentary individuals from different formulae.

It is also widely recognised that males and females exhibit differences in fat distribution. This sexual dimorphism appears at puberty and is most marked in early adulthood. The android distribution is characterised by a pattern where excess fat preferentially accumulates on the torso, with the effect that the waist profile is 'filled in'. By contrast, the gynoid distribution is characterised by fat accumulation in the gluto-femoral regions, and a clear waist profile is preserved. These have historically been referred to as the 'apple' and 'pear' shapes, which describe these generalised distribution. The importance of phenotypic variation and its application to health, attractiveness and body image are considered in Chapter 4.

In physical activity and sport, males generally outperform females, and there may be a number of reasons for this. It is possible to attribute the body to a simple biomechanical model, first by suggesting that it comprises productive mass (muscles, bone, nerve tissue, blood, essential regulatory organs etc.) and ballast (excess fat) (Carter, 1985). If we consider the world records held by women and men in the same event, we generally observe a narrowing of the performance difference in recent decades. Such a difference across all competitive running distances appears to vary between about 8 and 11 per cent. We could reasonably expect this to correspond closely to the composition difference relating to fat or muscle between the two, although such data are not in the public domain. However, questions could be raised with respect to early records resulting from very small numbers of participants, and the possibility that some could have been set in an era when athletes have undergone illegal performance enhancement via undetected banned substances. Nevertheless, the observation that performance differences between males and females largely reflect body composition differences generates a dialogue involving physiology and biomechanics, and prompts the age-old question: will women ever equal or surpass men in sports performance? Although the most recent data from running may suggest otherwise, a longer time frame of consideration still suggests a convergence. In practice, biomechanical arguments underpinning enhanced performance reflect inertial mass, so there is a size-dependency as well. Endurance events such as the marathon in hotter environments might also favour smaller individuals as a function of a greater surface area to volume ratio for heat dissipation. In most situations involving men and women competing on equal terms, we can anticipate the morphological advantage bestowed on men to manifest in male dominance. One notable exception in 1967, was the UK 12-hour cycling race, when Beryl Burton rode 277 miles, beating a field of 99 men, and shattering the previous record (held by a male) by nearly five and a half miles. Such examples are extremely rare and men's superiority in strength events is normally considered to be greater than in endurance events. However, there are two sports in which females out perform males in absolute terms. These are long-distance open-water swimming, and free diving. Here the female morphology is better adapted to the task, in swimming by a greater fat content contributing both to buoyancy and insulating against heat loss. In free diving, the smaller active muscle mass of women and lower metabolism enables the available oxygen from a single breath to last longer, which in turn allows the athlete to dive deeper and endure the prolonged re-ascent.

Having set these definitions, frames of reference and applications for body composition in health and sport, we next need to examine in more detail how body composition is measured in Chapters 2 and 3.

References

Behnke, A.R. & Wilmore, J.H. (1974). *Evaluation and Regulation of Body Build and Composition*, Englewood Cliffs, NJ: Prentice Hall.

Björntorp, P. (1997). Body fat distribution, insulin resistance, and metabolic diseases, *Nutrition, 13*, 975–803.

Broom, I. & Rolland, C. (2010). Homo adipatus: a new species: weight management, treatment and prevention. In G. Tsichlia and A. Johnstone (Eds.) *Fat Matters: From Sociology to Science* (pp. 51–66). Keswick: M&K Publishing.

Carin-Levy, G., Greig, C.A., Lewis, S.J., Stewart, A., Young, A. & Mead G.E. (2008). The effect of different positions on anthropometric measurements and derived estimates of body composition. *International Journal of Body Composition Research, 6*, 17–20.

Carter, J.E.L. (1985). Morphological factors limiting human performance. In H.M. Eckert and D.H. Clarke (Eds.) *The Limits of Human Performance*, The American Academy of Physical Education Papers, No. 18 (pp. 106–117). Champaign, IL: Human Kinetics.

Clarys, J.P., Martin, A.D, Drinkwater, D.T. & Marfell-Jones, M.J. (1987). The skinfold: myth and reality. *Journal of Sports Sciences, 5*, 3–33.

Clarys, J.P., Provyn, S. & Marfell-Jones, M.J. (2005). Cadaver studies and their impact on the understanding of human adiposity. *Ergonomics, 48*, 1445–1461.

Drinkwater, D.T. & Ross, W.D. (1980). Anthropometric fractionation of body mass. In W. Ostyn, G. Beunen and J. Simons (Eds.) *Kinanthropometry II* (pp. 177–188). Baltimore, MD: University Park Press.

Durnin, J.V.G.A. & Womersley, J. (1974). Body fat assessed from total body density and its estimation from skinfold thickness: measurements on 481 mean and women aged from 16 to 72 years. *British Journal of Nutrition, 32*, 77–97.

Einhorn, T.A. (1996). The bone organ system: form and function. In R. Marcus, D. Feldman and J. Kelsey (Eds.) *Osteoporosis* (pp. 3–22). San Diego CA: Academic Press.

Eston, R.G., Hawes, M.R., Martin, A.D. and Reilly, T. (2009) Human body composition. In R. Eston and T. Reilly (Eds.) *Kinanthropometry and Exercise Physiology Laboratory Manual: Tests, Procedures and Data – Anthropometry*, 3rd Edition (pp. 3–53). London: Routledge.

Igoe, J.B. (Ed.) (1979). *Blakiston's Pocket Medical Dictionary*, 4th edition. New York: McGraw-Hill.

Jackson, A.S. & Pollock, M.L. (1978). Generalized equations for predicting body density of men. *British Journal of Nutrition, 40*, 497–504.

Jackson, A.S., Pollock, M.L. & Ward, A. (1980). Generalized equations for predicting body density of women. *Medicine and Science in Sports and Exercise, 12*, 175–182.

Lauderdale, D.S. & Rathouz, P.J. (1999). Evidence of environmental suppression of familial resemblance: height among US Civil War brothers. *Annals of Human Biology, 26*, 413–426.

Martin, A.D., Spenst, L.F., Drinkwater, D.T. & Clarys, J.P. (1990). Anthropometric estimation of muscle mass in men. *Medicine and Science in Sports and Exercise, 22*, 729–733.

Matiegka, J. (1921). The testing of physical efficiency. *American Journal of Physical Anthropology, 4*, 223–230.

Nindl, B.C., Friedl, K.E., Marchitelli, L.J., Shippee, R.L., Thomas, C.D. & Patton, J.F. (1996). Regional fat placement in physically fit males and changes with weight loss. *Medicine and Science in Sports and Exercise, 28*, 786–793.

Rognum, T.O., Rodahl, K. & Opstad, P.K. (1982). Regional differences in the lipolytic response of the subcutaneous fat depots to prolonged exercise and severe energy deficiency. *European Journal of Applied Physiology, 49*, 401–408.

Salmon, J., Bauman, A., Crawford, D., Timperio, A. & Owen, N. (2000). The association between television viewing and overweight among Australian adults participating in varying levels of leisure-time physical activity. *International Journal of Obesity and Related Metabolic Disorders, 24*, 600–606.

Silventoinen, K. (2003). Determinants of variation in adult body height. *Journal of Biosocial Science, 35*, 263–285.

Stewart, A.D. (2010). Kinanthropometry and body composition: a natural home for 3D photonic scanning. *Journal of Sports Sciences, 28,* 455–457.

Tyrrell, A.R., Reilly, T. & Troup J.D.G. (1985). Circadian variation in stature and the effects of spinal loading. *Spine, 10,* 161–164.

Wang, Z.M., Pierson, R.N.J. & Heymsfield, S.B. (1992). The five level model: a new approach to organizing body composition research. *American Journal of Clinical Nutrition, 56,* 19–28.

2

LABORATORY METHODS OF BODY COMPOSITION ANALYSIS

Catherine Rolland

This chapter will cover:

2.1 Cadaver analysis

In the initial stages of body composition analysis, cadavers were analysed and later used as a criterion method for validating developing methods which could be used in live subjects. Cadavers have been analysed chemically and anatomically. The chemical approach has allowed the measurement of fat, protein and minerals while the anatomical approach has allowed the determination of the gross tissue weight for different parts of the body separated by dissection. Most information available today is based on analyses performed in the mid–1900s (Matiegka, 1921; Widdowson, McCance & Spray, 1951). This method represents the only truly accurate measurement of composition because of the capability for chemical assessment of dissectible tissue. The mass of these tissues collectively equals that of the fresh cadaver after evaporation of body fluids during the dissection process.

The use of cadaver analysis has been essential for comparison and validation of indirect methods of assessing body composition. In 1984, in a collaboration between a Belgian and a Canadian group, an analysis of 25 cadavers was carried out to provide normative data on the weights and densities of the different body compartments (i.e. skin, adipose tissue, muscle, bone and vital organs) as well as validating indirect methods for the *in vivo* estimation of body composition and to provide new models for the assessment of body composition (Clarys, Martin & Drinkwater, 1984). The outcomes for these validation studies (referred to as the Brussels Cadaver Study) resulted in the conclusion that there were no satisfactory methods for the *in vivo* estimation of muscle, bone and adipose tissue weights in humans, due to a very small amount of direct data available. In 1990, however, the research group was able to develop acceptable prediction equations for estimating muscle mass based on cadaver analysis (Martin, Spenst, Drinkwater & Clarys, 1990).

Today we have access to a number of different laboratory methods, each with their advantages and limitations. These are used to create multiple compartment models which are now considered to be the most accurate as they include measurements of body composition at several levels ranging from the atomic to the whole-body level. Multi-component methods, however, are costly and time consuming, hence the need for simpler and more rapidly used methods of acceptable accuracy.

2.2 Underwater weighing (densitometry)

Underwater weighing was long considered as a criterion method for estimating percentage body fat. Modern hydrodensitometry systems consist of a scale and a large heated tank of water (commonly 35–37°C). The participant exhales maximally, while totally immersed and body weight is then recorded. This is repeated at least five times and the highest value is used directly, or alternatively the mean of the highest two or three readings.

Underwater weighing is based on the principles of Archimedes (287–212 BC) where the specific gravity of an object is hypothesised to be the ratio of its mass to the mass of an equal volume of water where:

$$\text{Specific gravity} = \frac{\text{Weight in air}}{(\text{weight in air} - \text{weight in water})}$$

This calculation can be applied for the determination of body volume and body density through water submersion where the loss of weight in water (weight in air - weight in water) equals the weight of displaced water. The water displaced represents a known volume because the density of water is known and constant at different temperatures, provided in Table 2.1.

Theoretically, underwater weighing can be performed in any still water of adequate depth, for instance a swimming pool. In practice, the most common set-up is a specialised small water tank and a seat suspended on cables attached to a load cell which allows the immersion of the participant into the tank. Prior to measuring, the participants are weighed in air wearing swimwear before entering

TABLE 2.1 Water density at different temperatures

Water temperature (°C)	Water density (g/cm³)
38	0.993
35	0.994
31	0.995
28	0.996
25	0.997

the tank and dislodging air bubbles on the skin surface. Participants are required to expel as much air as possible from their lungs during complete submersion and are then weighed, as illustrated in Figure 2.1.

Residual lung volume is then calculated – most commonly with the participant in the tank with the head above the water level. Residual air trapped inside the body (lungs, gastro-intestinal tract) is highly buoyant, and is not part of the body, and therefore needs to be adjusted for. Hence the density equation needs to account for this:

$$\text{Body Density } (D_b) = \frac{\text{weight in air (kg)}}{[(\text{weight in air (kg)} - \text{weight in water (kg)}) / \text{Density of water}] - \text{trapped air (l)}}$$

(Trapped air comprises the sum of measured residual volume, and gut gas (most commonly assumed to be 0.1 l).)

Body mass can be divided into its fat (f_{fat}) and fat-free (f_{FFM}) fractions such that

$$1 / D_b = f_{fat} / D_{fat} + f_{FFM} / D_{FFM}$$

where D_{fat} and D_{FFM} are the densities for the fat and fat free mass compartments, respectively (Ellis, 2000).

Residual lung volume can be predicted from gender, age and stature, but can also be measured directly through oxygen dilution, helium dilution or nitrogen washout. For oxygen dilution, the individual takes six deep breaths of a known quantity of pure oxygen (commonly using an anaesthetic bag with exactly 3 l), beginning and ending with complete expiration (Wilmore, Vodak, Parr, Girandola & Billing, 1980).

For nitrogen washout:

$$RV = \frac{VO_2 \times FEN_2}{(0.798 - FEN_2)} - DS \times CF$$

(Where VO_2 is measured into an anaesthetic bag; FEN_2 is the fraction of N_2 at equilibrium $[100 - (\%O_2 + \%CO_2)] / 100$ DS is dead space of mouthpiece and valve; CF is the correction factor for body temperature and pressure, saturated (BTPS) to adjust the measured gas volume to that of the lung.

Percentage body fat can be calculated using simple equations such as the Siri (1956) or the Brozek, Frande, Anderson & Keys (1963) equations.

$$\% \text{ fat (Siri)} = [(4.95 / Db) - 4.50] \times 100$$

$$\% \text{ fat (Brozek et al.)} = [(4.57 / Db) - 4.142] \times 100$$

The Siri and the Brozek et al. equations are based on the two-compartment model, suggesting that the body is composed of fat mass and fat-free mass (FFM; comprising bone, water and other lean tissues). This is somewhat simplistic as fat-free mass composition has been shown to vary considerably with age, gender, ethnicity and exercise. Nevertheless, this approach is highly reproducible to within 1% for individuals. More complex equations can also be used for calculating percentage body fat from body density based on four compartment models, which take account of the variation in FFM constituents.

Underwater weighing methods were developed to determine body fat as a percentage of total body mass. Due to variations in body hydration, protein and mineral content, however, it has been estimated that a total cumulative error for 3–4 per cent can result when determining the percentage body fat of an individual. Without a correction factor to account for this variation, it is suggested that densitometry should not be used as a reference method for heterogeneous populations (Ellis, 2000).

A number of assumptions need to be made for calculating body density and percentage body fat. It is assumed that the separate densities of the body components are cumulative (i.e. can be arithmetically combined according to their proportions to form the overall body density), that the density of body constituents are constant

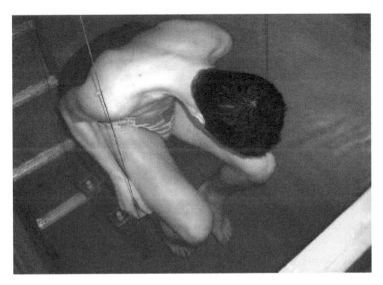

FIGURE 2.1 The measurement of underwater weight.

between individuals; that the proportions of the constituents of the fat-free mass are constant from person to person; that a subject being measured differs from a reference body only in fat content; and that buoyant gas at the time of underwater weighing can be estimated. Unfortunately, none of these assumptions can be fully justified. It is further assumed that the density of fat remains constant, however, there is reason to believe that there may be variations of fat density in relation to gender, ethnicity, growth, sexual maturation, ageing, physical activity, and disease (Ellis, 2000).

There are also a number of limitations with underwater weighing. First, the individual being measured needs to be comfortable to be immersed in the water while sustaining a maximal exhalation. In addition, for the measurements to be accurate, the individual has to have recovered from previous exercise, to be fasted, fully hydrated and voided. The water in the tank needs to be stirred/mixed to ensure that the water does not stratify and that temperature (and therefore density) of the water remains constant. In theory, underwater weighing is capable of providing body density estimates on very large individuals, however, not all obese patients are able to participate in this procedure which requires climbing steps, descending into a tank of water and holding their breath under water at maximal exhalation. However, for suitably water-confident individuals the procedure need not be limited to specialist laboratory settings and can be performed in swimming or hydrotherapy pools.

Although underwater weighing has historically been considered the gold standard body composition estimate, it may be impractical to implement in most clinical and research settings.

2.3 Air displacement plethysmography

Air displacement plethysmography (ADP) is a rapid, comfortable, non-invasive and safe way of measuring body volume and percentage body fat. Unlike several other methods for assessing body volume, ADP is also able to accommodate various groups of people, including children, obese (although limited in individuals with extreme morbid obesity to below a body mass index (BMI) of $50 \, kg.m^{-2}$), elderly and disabled persons.

This method uses similar fundamental principles to hydrodensitometry where body volume is measured within a known capsule volume and the air pressure difference is detected following breathing. Since the 1990s there has been a commercially available machine for ADP called the BodPod (COSMED, Rome, Italy). The system consists of two linked but separate chambers: one serving as a reference volume and the other for the participant. The individual is required to wear close-fitting clothing and a swim cap to minimise trapped air and to remove all jewellery. The participant is required to sit in the measuring chamber and to remain still during the measurement. Once the door is closed and sealed, the pressure increases slightly, and a diaphragm separating the two chambers oscillates which alters the pressure and volume in each. The ratio of the pressures is a measure of the test chamber volume, which is calibrated by a known volume of 50 litres before measuring an individual. The air in the chamber is allowed to compress and expand adiabatically (without heat gain or loss) making use of Poisson's Law which states that the ratio of the volumes of the test and reference chambers is equal to the ratio of the pressure amplitudes following perturbation. The relationship of pressure versus volume, at a fixed temperature, is used to calculate the volume of the participant in the measuring chamber as illustrated in Figure 2.2.

When carrying out the measurement, one needs to account for temperature change, gas composition (CO_2 and O_2) as well as isothermal versus adiabatic conditions. There is also a need to account for clothing, hair, body surface area and thoracic gas volume. Moisture on the skin as well as hair alters the correction for compressibility of air next to the body surface, leading to an underestimation of percentage body fat.

When measuring body volume by means of ADP, it is assumed that this is taking place in adiabatic conditions. There are, however, a number of potential sources of error due to the presence of isothermal air, the volume of which can be compressed 40 per cent more than adiabatic air. The sources of isothermal air include air trapped in the hair, air in the lungs, air close to the skin and air trapped in clothing. These sources of isothermal air are minimised by ensuring that the individual being measured is wearing a swim cap, by measuring air in the lungs and correcting for it, and by ensuring participants either wear a tight fitting swim suit or Lycra shorts. Air close to the skin is also corrected for automatically by the software by calculating a surface area artefact (SAA) based on an estimation of body surface area calculated from body mass and stature. Inaccuracies in these, whether from biological variation in stature and mass, or the formula used to predict surface area will thus contribute to error in the calculation of percentage body fat because of inappropriate estimates of SAA.

A failure to account and correct for sources of isothermal air results in an underestimation of body volume. The importance of wearing appropriate clothing during ADP using the BodPod was investigated by Peeters & Claessens (2009). They investigated the potential for measuring individuals in a public setting (for example a gym) wearing sports apparel. Their findings demonstrated not only that this approach resulted in a significant underestimation of body volume, overestimation of body density, underestimation of body fat but that these measurements had poor test-retest reliability even if the individuals were wearing exactly the same clothing for their repeat measurements. There was also a significant trend of increasing error as body density increases. Interestingly, these researchers more recently demonstrated that even wearing different types of swim caps can result in significantly different body measurement (Peeters & Claessens, 2010). Their results demonstrated that Lycra swim caps do not compress the scalp hair adequately when compared to a silicon cap, not fully eliminating the effect of isothermal air trapped in scalp hair and therefore resulting in and underestimation of body volume.

Other conditions that need to be met for the accurate use of the BodPod system are that the equipment should ideally be in a room of its own, in specific temperature and humidity ranges that do not alter substantially. Changes in pressure due to windows, doors shutting and other movements in the building may affect the

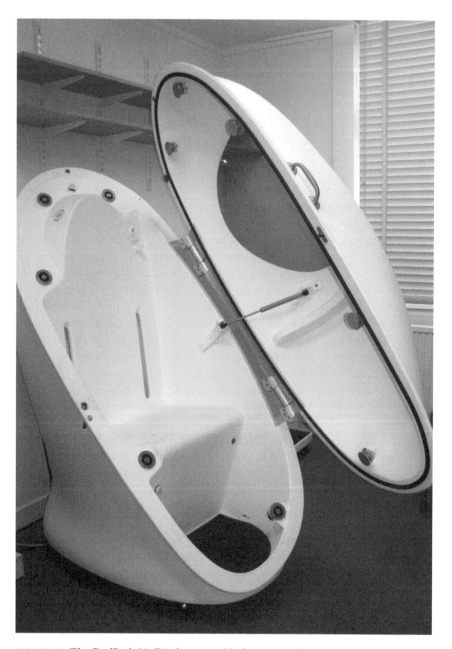

FIGURE 2.2 The BodPod Air Displacement Plethysmograph.

validity of the measurements, although avoiding these may be hard to achieve in practice. It is also essential that the participant remains still and breathes regularly because irregular tidal breathing (e.g. yawning, throat clearing, coughing, laughing or breath-holding) will jeopardise the accuracy of the measurement.

Although the BodPod is a system that is straightforward to use and is reliable, there remain some limitations in the use of this approach. Individuals who are either very tall or very large may find it difficult to fit in the BodPod. The equipment is still to be validated for these and other groups of interest (e.g. sufferers of certain disease conditions, disabled individuals or pregnant women). In addition, in some instances individuals can experience claustrophobia while inside the BodPod. Despite these limitations, ADP is a promising method for percentage body fat estimation and future work should be done to validate its use in different populations and with larger numbers of participants.

2.4 Isotope dilution methods

Isotope dilution can be used to assess body composition through the use of tracers. Their use is based on the assumption that the volume of a compartment is equal to the ratio of the dose of a tracer/concentration in that body compartment within a short time after the dose is administered (Ellis, 2000). The tracer can either be administered orally or intravenously. To measure the tracer, usually two body fluids are collected (e.g. saliva, urine or blood). An initial body fluid collection would be carried out followed by the administration of the tracer. This would provide a background level of the tracer before administration. The body fluid would then be collected again after a pre-determined time for the penetration of the tracer within the compartment of interest, and for equilibrium to be reached. If a significant amount of tracer is excreted before equilibrium is reached, then a cumulative urine sample (up to 24 hours) may be collected to adjust dose estimate, or alternatively, several blood samples can be collected and the tracer content can be extrapolated to time zero.

When assessing body composition by means of a tracer, a number of assumptions are made. The first assumption is that the tracer is equally distributed only in the exchangeable pool (i.e. the body fluids in which the tracer is in a dynamic state). The second assumption is that the tracer is equally distributed within this pool. Third, that the tracer is not metabolised during the equilibration time; and fourth, that the tracer equilibrium is achieved relatively rapidly. Any breach of these assumptions requires the adjustment of the ratio of administered dose of tracer to fluid concentration.

The measurement of total body water (TBW) allows for the determination of FFM because of the differential hydration status of fat and FFM, since FFM contains approximately 73 per cent water (although this varies with age) and fat mass contains very little water. With TBW and the hydration coefficient, FFM can be estimated. Isotopes of oxygen and hydrogen are introduced into the body as labelled water. The molecules diffuse through the body and equilibrate with the body water. The extent to which the isotope concentration has been diluted indicates the quantity of water in the body.

For TBW, the most direct *in vivo* measurement is based on the dilution principle using tracer dose of labelled water (Tritium (^{3}H), deuterium (D_2O) or oxygen–18 (^{18}O). This method requires the collection of two body fluids with a sampling pre-dose and the second collection after an equilibration time of two to three hours. A larger body water pool would be indicated by a lower isotope concentration.

For extracellular water (ECW) measurement, the basic dilution techniques are the same as for TBW. The difference, however, lies in the administration and collection. The tracer is added to the water and the body fluid usually sampled is plasma. Non-radioactive bromine is the most commonly used tracer. The tracer is administered orally with a second plasma sample collected approximately three to four hours later.

Intracellular water volume can be measured using the dilution of radioactive potassium (^{42}K), but this tracer is short lived and is no longer commercially available. Today, an oral dose of D_2O and bromine is more commonly used from which TBW and ECW are determined and intracellular water (ICW) can then be calculated by subtracting the ECW from the TBW. Thus, calculating ICW involves the cumulative error of the measurements for TBW and ECW.

The method of analysis is dependent on the choice of tracer. ^{3}H is measured by radioactive beta-counting; ^{18}O is measured by mass spectroscopy; D_2O is measured by infrared absorption, gas chromatography or mass spectroscopy and bromine is measured by high pressure liquid chromatography, X-ray fluorescence, spectrophotometry or mass spectrometry. When determining the tracer to be utilised, it is important to note that ^{18}O is very expensive, and that ^{3}H is cheap but radioactive. Also, background levels are important when D_2O or ^{18}O are used because these occur naturally in the body, while natural levels of ^{3}H in the body are very low. The dose of the tracer injected is dependent on the mass of the participant and time of body fluid collection. This method of measuring percentage body fat is now generally used as part of multi-compartment models against which cheaper and more practical methods of assessment can be compared (Ellis, 2000).

2.5 Medical imaging methods

There are a number of medical imaging techniques available. These include whole body potassium, computed tomography, magnetic resonance imaging and ultrasound. Medical imaging methods use different physical properties to determine internal dimensions and volumes. Most medical imaging methods are used for diagnostics, although they can be adapted for body composition.

Total body potassium (TBK)

Potassium occurs naturally in the body, and because of this a background value needs to be established. The radioactive isotope ^{40}K makes up ~0.012 per cent of natural potassium in the body and emits high-energy gamma (γ) rays of 1.46 MeV. More than 50 per cent of these rays will exit the body where they can be externally measured. To do this safely and accurately requires (1) γ-ray detectors with high energy resolution and efficiency; (2) adequate shielding around the subject and detectors to reduce the background levels; and (3) a means of identifying and recording the 1.46 MeV γ-ray of the ^{40}K (Ellis, 2000). The subject is placed in a supine position under sodium iodide detectors within a room constructed of a steel shield. Steel itself has contained much higher levels of background activity since the nuclear events of Hiroshima and Nagasaki, and the subsequent nuclear testing in Pacific atolls in the 1950s. As a result, TBK shields are frequently made from radiation-free steel salvaged from ships built before the Second World War, and ^{40}K is recorded as the supine participant slowly passes beneath the detectors to determine the TBK. Although it had been previously assumed that the K fraction in FFM was fairly constant, values ranging from 52–68 meq/kg are reported in Ellis (2000) justifying caution when it is used to estimate FFM or body cell mass. With the development of alternative methods, TBK has become less routine in body composition research, but is still used in occupational health settings to assess radiation exposure for workers in the nuclear industry.

In vivo neutron activation (IVNA)

Controlled neutron irradiation transforms atoms of a chemical element from their ground state to the next nuclear state. In a fraction of a nano-second, the nucleus descends to its ground state again, resulting in the release of γ-rays which have element-specific energies. If, following neutron capture, the atom is altered to a radioactive isotope, the energy will decay over time with a known half-life. Controlled neutron beams can be of varying energies where rapidly moving neutrons are optimal for tissue penetration, however, most IVNA methods rely on low energy (or thermal) neutrons. The energies for a number of elements that occur in the body (i.e. H, C, N, O, Na, Ca, P and Cl) can be quantified using this method although IVNA is most frequently used to measure total body calcium and total body nitrogen. Different elements require different radiation doses for quantification. For example, nitrogen measurement requires a relatively low dose (< 0.3 mSv) while calcium measurements require a much larger dose (> 3 mSv) (Ellis, 2000). The main drawbacks of IVNA is primarily the radiation dose associated with it and, with a relative scarcity of facilities, there is also a lack of standardisation between different instrument designs for the measurement of IVNA.

Computed tomography

Computed axial tomography (CAT or CT) scans use a high dose of ionising radiation in the form of X-rays to image a variety of tissues in the body. The X-ray beam is passed through the body and measured by detectors positioned on the far side of the subject. The X-ray source and detector assembly is rotated as a single unit around the body. Although CT is acquired in the axial plane, coronal and sagittal images can be produced by computer reconstruction. Radiocontrast agents are often used with CT for enhanced delineation of anatomical structures.

Both CT and magnetic resonance imaging (MRI) images are composed of pixels, which are usually 1 mm × 1 mm and have a third dimension relating to slice thickness. Volume elements are referred to as voxels which have a grey scale that provides image contrast and reflects tissue composition. Although CT images appear similar to those of MRI, the grey scale contrast indicating different tissues is reversed. As a method, CT is highly accurate and precise for measurement, but this comes at the expense of a high radiation dose (i.e. ~1-21 mSv per examination using a single-slice spiral CT depending on the site being assessed (Brix et al., 2003).

Magnetic resonance imaging (MRI)

Hydrogen nuclei (protons) are abundant in living tissues and have magnetic moments which result in them acting as small magnets. These magnetic moments are usually random and cancel each other out, but when subjected to the external magnet of a MRI scanner, the protons have a high affinity for alignment with the magnetic field. The frequency at which the nuclei will change orientation (relative to the direction of the magnetic field) is called the Larmor frequency. When radiofrequency (RF) energy, at the Larmor frequency, is applied perpendicular to the direction of the magnetic field, the nuclei will absorb the energy and change alignment. When the applied RF signal is turned off, the stored energy is released as an induced RF signal when the nuclei resume their original positions. Parameters of this induced signal are manipulated by the MRI software to produce images characterising specific tissues

Since adipose and lean tissue do not vary greatly in hydrogen densities, to enhance the imaging contrast between lean and fat tissue, another property of the nuclei, the relaxation time (T1 in ms) is also used. Relaxation time refers to the time it takes for the nuclei to release the RF-induced energy and return to a random configuration. T1 for protons in fat is considerably shorter than that for protons in water (Ellis, 2000).

To obtain a whole body image by MRI, a series of multiple scans along the length of the body are required. This procedure can take 30 minutes or longer, by acquiring blocks of images which are subsequently joined together. Figure 2.3 depicts an abdominal cross-section measured at the umbilicus. MRI has been validated by cadaver analysis and is very useful for body composition as it has the potential for measuring visceral and subcutaneous adipose tissue (VAT and SAT respectively) compartments separately. Most of the literature on MRI scanning involves the supine body, but more recently, positional MRI enables the measurement to be acquired in any orientation, which has provided valuable insight into structural adjustments arising from postural factors relating to the plasticity of tissues or fluid movement within the body, or differential loading of the spine in different orientations.

Although both CT and MRI generate accurate total and regional body volumes and dimensions, these procedures are expensive and neither is risk free for the subject. Neither method is widely used for body composition purposes due to their high cost and, in the case of CT, high radiation exposure. They remain expensive for routine use, but can validate other more affordable methods.

Ultrasound scanning is a further type of medical imaging that has been used routinely for safe pre-natal scans for the delineation of structures in a growing foetus. It has also been used to assess superficial and deep adipose tissue in other clinical settings. More recently, advances have enabled this technology to become portable and, as a result, it is described in Chapter 3.

Both CT and MRI are considered to be sophisticated laboratory body composition methods. However, neither of these methods has been validated for the assessment of total body fat against a robust method such as the four-compartment method approach. More commonly, MRI and CT total body composition is determined by acquiring slices at specific anatomical locations and interpolating between these slices to determine volumes using a geometric model based on either a parallel trapezium or truncated cone. Tissue volumes are then related to mass via assumed densities.

Some studies have attempted to validate CT and MRI by comparison with cadavers (Rössner et al., 1990; Mitsiopoulos et al., 1998) but only do so for certain sections of the body (e.g. subcutaneous and visceral adipose tissue in the abdomen, and subcutaneous adipose tissue in arms and legs). Total percentage body fat

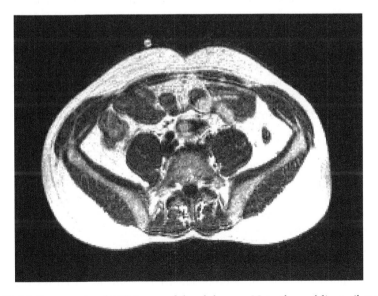

FIGURE 2.3 Cross sectional MRI scan of the abdomen. Note the cod liver oil capsule used to landmark the level of the umbilicus.

determined by MRI was compared to percentage body fat by underwater weighing (UWW) (Sohlström, Wahlund & Forsum, 1993), however, as discussed above, the limitations of UWW preclude its use as a valid reference for quantifying accuracy. This underscores the need to assess the true accuracy of CT and MRI for the determination of total percentage body fat compared to the four-compartment model, if it is to be used for total percentage fat determination. More commonly, both techniques are used for diagnostics, and composition of specified regions, and not the whole body.

2.6 Dual X-ray absorptiometry

Dual X-ray absorptiometry (DXA) (sometimes called dual-energy X-ray absorptiometry) was developed from single photon absorptiometry using Iodine-125 on the proximal and distal ulna. This was replaced with dual photon absorptiometry using Gadolinium-153. This produces gamma emissions at 44 and 100 keV which enabled estimates of bone mineral density. DXA emerged when radioactive isotopes were replaced with an X-ray source. The filtered beam resulted in high and low energies which are absorbed to differing extents according to the tissue characteristics. Absorption/attenuation characteristics can be measured using chemicals and tissue equivalents to simulate the human body.

When a photon source is directed at one side of an object, the intensity of the beam at the other side is determined by the object's thickness, density and chemical composition. This phenomenon is referred to as attenuation – and this enables a DXA scan to produce a composition map of the scanned area of the supine body. A measurement is made of the attenuation of the X-ray beam at both energies, at every point in the scanned area using the ratio of attenuation of the beam at the two energies – the R value. With this, different components of the body are grouped into three different categories by their X-ray attenuation properties, calibrated against tissue-equivalent standards. Attenuation properties of different tissues vary according to the differing atomic masses of the elements they contain. Bone mineral contains calcium and phosphorous in large quantities while lean soft tissue contains small quantities of potassium, chlorine, sulphur, calcium and iron, mostly as electrolytes. Fat, however, contains only hydrogen, carbon and oxygen.

When measuring bone mineral density, bone mass is referred to as bone mineral content (BMC). Bone mineral density (BMD), however, is the quantity of bone mass per unit area, and is therefore an areal density in $g.cm^{-2}$. Bone area is calculated as the area of pixels containing bone.

For soft tissue composition assessment (i.e. determining fat and fat-free soft tissue mass), at established energies of 40 and 70 KeV, fat produces an attenuation coefficient of 1.18 (R_f) and 1.399 for fat free soft tissue (R_l). Given the consistency between subjects of these, the ratio of attenuation at the lower energy relative to the higher energy soft tissue (R_{st}) is a function of the proportion of fat (R_f) and fat free soft tissue (R_l) in each pixel:

$$\text{Lean fraction } L_f = [R_{st} - R_f] / [R_1 - R_f]$$

Where soft tissue and bone are layered, if the relative intensity of the photon beam can be measured, and the mass attenuation coefficients are known, estimates of the bone mass and overlying soft tissue mass can be calculated.

Although DXA does not provide three independent measurements, values for three different body composition tissues are calculated (bone mineral content (BMC), fat-free soft tissue mass and fat mass). To obtain these values, it is assumed that the composition of the soft tissue layer overlying the bone has the same fat-to-lean ratio as that for non-bone pixels in the same scan region (Ellis, 2000). Note that the use of 'lean' tissue can be misleading, because elsewhere it is defined as including essential lipids. Fat-free mass and fat-free soft tissue mass (which excludes BMC) are less ambiguous.

It is also possible to use DXA to estimate muscle mass. The mass of appendicular fat-free soft tissue (AFFST) can be estimated from DXA but muscle mass predictions rely on the assumption that all non-fat and non-bone tissue is muscle mass, and that the appendicular and torso muscle occur in a known ratio. In reality, AFFST's largest proportion comprises skeletal muscle, but it also comprises skin, connective tissue and the lean portion of adipose tissue. This assumption of AFFST equating to muscle should be reasonably accurate in the arms, legs, and regions in between joints where the amount of tendons and cartilage are small (Visser, Fuerst, Lang, Salamone & Harris, 1999). A number of models have been developed to determine skeletal muscle mass based on measurements of AFFST, but often require adjustments for age and gender which will have an effect on AFFST. The models available need to be validated across different populations, but still provide an important alternative to CT and MRI for the assessment of muscle mass.

The use of DXA for determining composition requires us to make a number of assumptions. It is assumed that body tissues are represented by attenuation coefficients; soft tissue composition in pixels containing bone can be estimated from neighbouring pixels according to the fat distribution model; and that anterior-posterior thickness does not affect measurements. It has been reported that DXA significantly underestimates percent body fat in lean individuals and overestimates fat in the obese (LaForgia, Dollman, Dale, Withers & Hill, 2009). Although there is a trend for DXA to progressively underestimate percent body fat of leaner individuals, which could be accounted for using correction factors, in the obese there appears to be no systematic bias. Previous work using DXA found that large errors in percentage body fat were associated with increasing tissue thickness, where the thicker the tissue under analysis, the greater the degree of 'beam hardening' which results in greater attenuation of the lower energy X-rays. The results from LaForgia et al. (2009) suggested that the precision of estimating percentage body fat using DXA remains questionable. Due to this, they proposed that DXA may be suitable for providing acceptable descriptive cross-sectional body composition data for obese cohorts but is less suitable for providing accurate measures at the individual level.

As highlighted previously, DXA is unable to measure soft tissue overlying the bone and assumes that the soft tissue adjacent to the bone has the same tissue composition as the soft tissue overlying the bone. This assumption may cause a greater error associated with all soft tissue measurements in muscular athletes due to larger variations of soft tissue over bone associated with various distributions of muscle and fat.

There are also a number of practical issues that need to be considered with DXA. These include X-ray dosage (and obtaining ethics permission and consent for the measurement), ensuring that the individual to be measured is not pregnant, as well as practical difficulties for participants fitting on the equipment in relation to stature, body size (for obese individuals and larger athletes). In addition, clothing, jewellery, calcified tissue, metal implants and movement all affect measurement.

The DXA scanning approach, using the older pencil beam or newer fan beam configurations, remains a very useful tool for the assessment of body composition, as the resultant radiation exposure from a whole body scan is relatively minor (depending on the machine model) and is comparable to the unavoidable daily background radiation. This has made it a more acceptable method of determining body composition in at-risk groups including children. Dual X-ray absorptiometry is also useful when investigating the effects of disability on body composition where changes in bone mineral density and lean-tissue hydration are evident, and where the presence of artefacts such as surgical implants can be adjusted for. But DXA scanning is not without its limitations. Scans are stable for normal ranges of adiposity and size (up to 25 cm thick), but not as accurate for larger individuals where the error is magnified. Bone data are altered via measurement artefacts in a person with changing adiposity, while clothing and gut content are included in the calculations for fat free soft tissue/fat. Significant variation is observed in measurement for the same individual using different manufacturers' instruments (Ellis, 2000). Disparities in potential error exist among different DXA machines and models, making comparisons between investigations difficult and underscoring the need for standardisation of the procedures. Protein mass is not specifically measured and therefore, the estimate for the lean mass using DXA can vary from the true protein mass.

Errors in estimating percentage body fat in women due to fluctuations in total body water through various stages of menstrual cycle have also been reported and there is evidence to suggest that DXA may not be appropriate for estimating percentage body fat in Caucasian female athletes (Moon et al., 2009). Finally, DXA scanning can be limited for very obese individuals where body size 'allowance' is limited by the scan area for the DXA machine. More recently, the GE Healthcare Lunar iDXA has become available which has a scanning bed which can withstand greater weights and provides a larger scanning width as well as producing higher resolution images. In addition, this equipment allows one side of the scanning table to be extended to allow for half-body scans of extremely large individuals. This new equipment appears to provide good precision for total body measurements of body composition and fat distribution (Hind, Olroyd & Truscott, 2011) and accurate measurement of non-bone lean and fat masses, and percentage body fat in obese adults (Rothney, Brychta, Schaefer, Chen & Skarulis, 2009) using half-body scans.

Despite the limitations and assumptions required, DXA scans can be performed within minutes and can provide immediate results with region specific composition data via computer software. Future work for the development of DXA scanning would require precision studies for a variety of populations (e.g. children, the obese, athletes or the disabled). The unique ability for DXA to estimate regional composition means that it has considerable potential for future body composition research. Pixel size and regional boundary placement during analysis invariably mean that regional precision, especially in the arms, is poorer than that of the whole body. In view of the recognised differences between different manufacturers' scanners and software, and the limited success of previous standardisation attempts, more work needs to be undertaken to standardise DXA results between different systems.

2.7 3D photonic scanning

Three-dimensional photonic imaging was developed in the late 1950s from stereo photogrammetry and was subsequently developed as a technology for whole-body surface measurements in humans. Several different models of scanners have been developed and improved on over the years, enhancing the data density and the speed of acquisition for measurement to ~10s, generating values for regional body volumes and dimensions as well as for total body volume. Measurements and ratios of different body girths such as waist-hip or waist-chest ratio can provide important information about weight distribution. This can be done by measuring skin folds and anthropometry, but multiple manual measurements can be time-consuming, supporting the potential usefulness of three-dimensional photonic scanning (3DPS). Also, manual anthropometric measurements and 3DPS may not be directly equivalent as hand-held tape measures on the skin surface, even although they aim not to indent the skin, may do so to a limited extent in order to locate the tape itself and hence compresses the circumference being measured, which is not an issue for 3DPS.

Three-dimensional laser imaging is a non-invasive optical method that uses high speed digital cameras and trigonometric principles to detect the actual position of laser-light points projected onto the surface of an object and reflected to cameras. Approaches to 3D body scanning are described in more detail in Chapter 4. Irrespective of which shape capture modality is adopted, the participant is asked to wear close-fitting clothing to avoid obscuring the details of skin topography, and is required to stand still in a standard pose to minimise data shadow effect. The system calibration ensures lasers detect a stationary object in focus, but postural sway and breathing artefacts affect human scans. System software approaches involve automatic landmark recognition resulting in the generation of a 3D-body shell as well as values for standard dimensional analyses for girths, surface areas and volumes. These have enabled a range of body composition studies to have been undertaken, which are considered here.

In a study by Wang et al. (2006), a C9036-02 laser scanner (Hamamatsu Photonics, Hamamatsu, Japan) was compared to underwater weighing and anthropometry for validating the accuracy and reproducibility of total and regional body volumes and dimensions measurements in human subjects with a wide range of age, weight and body fatness and a commercially available mannequin. The protocol involved exhaling completely and maintaining a stationary posture for the scan duration. The body volumes and circumferences were significantly larger when measured using 3DPS when compared to underwater weighing, but there was no significant difference in percentage body fat when comparing the two methods. Despite volumes being greater with 3DPS, these differences were considered to be small and not necessarily clinically significant. However, scientifically, the finding bears closer scrutiny. Interestingly, age, sex and obesity did not affect the relationship between 3DPS and underwater weighing or tape measurements. In scientific (as opposed to clinical) terms, the lack of significant differences in the calculated percentage fat using the two-compartment method and the Siri equation, may indicate the inadequacy of this densitometric approach, as small volume differences have considerable influence over calculated density. In addition, the large age range (6–83 years) means the variability in the constituents of the FFM was likely to be considerable in this sample.

Measurements for the mannequin demonstrated the effect of clothing on 3DPS where the total body volume was significantly greater than that measured without clothing. This is simply due to the fact that the data points used to generate body volume when using 3DPS were reflected from the surface of the body or clothing. Overall, the authors concluded that 3DPS is an accurate and repeatable technique for measuring body volume and dimensions, provided participants wear suitable clothing.

An alternative light-based scanner was used for the UK National Sizing survey of adults (Size UK – Wells, Treleaven & Cole, 2007). The study used a cross section of these data to examine the relation between shape and BMI as well as to identify the interactive effects of age and sex on shape. The results suggested that the two main factors associated with BMI in men after adjustment for height are chest and waist, while in women, it is hip and bust girth. Hence, the genders differ in the body regions that appear to be most influential on BMI. The authors further suggest that chest in men but hips in women reflect physique, while waist in men and bust in women reflect fatness. In addition, the study highlighted the limitations of BMI in accounting for age-associated changes in the distribution of body mass, which the study showed to differ appreciably between genders. Associations of shape with age were significantly stronger in women than in men where shape implied a shift in fat toward the upper body with age for women. The development of a more android pattern of fat distribution with age in women and a lack of such an association in men, would suggest these changes are related to hormonal changes of female reproductive biology changing the strategy of energy deposition with age. As central obesity has been associated with increased risk of cardiovascular disease, this association of age with shape suggests a delay in the detrimental effect of centrally located fat in women which may contribute to the average greater life expectancy of women in industrialised countries. The study also found that differences in shape between genders were more pronounced in young adults and lessened with age.

Body scanning can acquire useful anthropometric measures for health research, without recourse to quantifying body fat. For instance, sagittal abdominal diameter has been found to be more strongly associated than waist circumference to visceral fat, which in turn is closely associated to cardiovascular risk while thigh girth has been found to have a protective effect for both heart disease and type 2 diabetes. Thus, 3DPS has potential for application in the prevention, classification and monitoring of diseases that are related to body shape, size or fatness such as growth and development, age, weight management, fitness management and pre- and postsurgical procedures. The association of different variables of shape with different diseases demonstrates the potential that monitoring changes in body shape has for informing clinicians about the risk of outcomes or even in response to diet, exercise or drug treatment in individual patients. Shape data have the potential to be developed into proxies for physiological markers of health and disease such as blood pressure, blood biochemistry and body fat distribution.

The technique of 3DPS has certain advantages over other body composition measures. The digital nature of data facilitates archiving and retrieval of scans, software allows superimposition of repeat scans to highlight changes. It is a safe and easy method for working with children, providing the child can stay still for the duration of the measurement. The technique also produces a three-dimensional topographical image which is more complete than a one-dimensional measurement like waist circumference and it remains cheaper than other imaging techniques such as CT or MRI and does not require specialised conditions or intensive technological support.

The main limitation of this technique is the requirement for the individual being measured to remain perfectly still for approximately 10–15 seconds (depending on the selected resolution and the model of 3D scanner) which would limit its use in the very young or the very ill. Similarly, body hair of sufficient density has been shown to increase the apparent size of body segments which may explain the differences between 3DPS and densitometrically determined volume.

Future work would require further validation to assess the repeatability and accuracy of the diverse measurements that can be obtained from photonic scans. Special attention should be given to posture, where a standard protocol for adopting and maintaining the stance during the measurement should be developed. Investigation of the relation between body shape and risk of morbidity and mortality and surrogate biomarkers for disease for different ethnicities is an important future research priority. Advances in computer graphics and scanning technology mean that 3DPS is likely to become more affordable and widespread for health and sports applications for body composition measurement in the future.

Many of the methods mentioned in this chapter require considerable research funding or clinical imperative before their costs can be justified. As a consequence, such laboratory techniques are beyond the means of many end users of body composition. This includes competitive athletes, and those following conditioning programmes, for whom less invasive and more affordable methods are warranted. For a review of current methods of body composition methods applied in sport, the reader is directed to Ackland et al. (2012) which highlights some of the issues involved with measuring athletes, and threats to the validity of the assumptions which this involves.

Multi-compartment models

As discussed above, each laboratory-based method is available for the estimation of body composition. Their attributes are summarised in Table 2.2. However, it is clear that each of these approaches is limited due to the assumptions associated with them. One way to overcome these limitations is through the use of multi-compartment models. As discussed in Chapter 1, Wang, Pierson & Heymsfield (1992) noted that body composition could be measured at the atomic, molecular, cellular, tissue and whole body level. The laboratory methods, which measure at these different levels of analysis, can be combined to form multi-compartment models which are now considered to be the gold standard for body composition estimation. Multi-compartment models have often been used for validating single methods of body composition estimates. The theory is that, by combining data from several laboratory methods into a multi-component model, the error associated with the assumptions for each individual method is reduced. Each measurement, however, needs to be compositionally independent of the other measurements. There are several published multi-compartment models available based on a number of different methodologies (e.g. body volume can be estimated either by air displacement plethysmography or underwater weighing). However, there is some discussion about the best multi-compartment model to use. The four-compartment model is currently very popular and is considered to be the criterion method for body composition is depicted in Figure 2.4. Nevertheless, it remains costly and time consuming which unfortunately limits its use at a clinical and research level.

TABLE 2.2 Summary of available lab techniques. Values are given for total body composition

Method	Measurement	Precision error	Accuracy	Advantage	Disadvantage
UWW	Density	±2%	96–97%	Applicability for larger individuals and children	Water immersion, fasting state, impractical
ADP	Density	±4.5%	>95%	Quick, comfortable, easy, non-invasive. Applicability for children, obese, elderly and disabled people	Stature and mass restrictions, claustrophobia, requirement of specific conditions for the measurement
CT	Areas/ volume	<1%	See Section 2.5	Generate accurate total and regional body volumes and dimensions	Radiation; high levels of training required; expensive
MRI	Areas/ volume	<2% for interobserver error	See Section 2.5	Generate accurate total and regional body volumes and dimensions	High levels of training required; very expensive
DXA	BMC, FM, FFM	±1%	97–99%	Quick; immediate results; applicability for children and disabled people	Radiation (although lower levels than CT); loses accuracy with increased fat mass; affected by hydration status
3D scanning	Surface area/ Volume	±0.4%	≥98%	Quick; non-invasive; safe	Requires individual to remain perfectly still, limiting its use in the very young or the very ill

CT: computed tomography; MRI: magnetic resonance imaging; DXA: dual X-ray absorptiometry; UWW: under water weighing; ADP: air displacement plethysmography; percentage accuracy is determined as (100 - % error), where the error is the percentage difference from the true value.
Note: The degree of automation versus manual region-of-interest identification in image analysis is highly influential on precision using MRI.

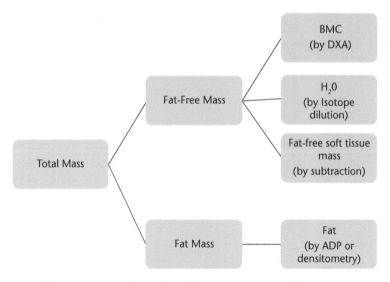

FIGURE 2.4 The most commonly used multi-compartment model.

BMC: bone mineral content; DXA: dual X-ray absorptiometry; ADP: air displacement plethysmography.

References

Ackland, T.R., Lohman, T.G., Sundgot-Borgen, J., Maughan, R.J., Meyer, N.L. Stewart, A.D. et al. (2012). Current status of body composition assessment in sport. *Sports Medicine* (advance-of-press ePublication), *42*, 227–249.

Brix, G., Nagel, H.D., Stamm, G., Veit, R., Lechel, U., Griebel, J. et al. (2003). Radiation exposure in multi-slice versus single-slice spiral CT: results of a nationwide survey. *European Radiology, 13*, 1979–1991.

Brozek, J., Grande, F., Anderson, J.T. & Keys, A. (1963). Densitometric analysis of body composition: revision of some quantitative assumptions. *Annals in the New York Academy of Sciences, 110*, 113–140.

Clarys, J.P., Martin, A.D. & Drinkwater, D.T. (1984) Gross tissue weights in the human body by cadaver dissection. *Human Biology, 56*, 459–473.

Ellis, K.J. (2000). Human body composition: *in vivo* methods. *Physiological Reviews, 80*, 649–680.

Hind, K., Oldroyd, B. & Truscott, J.G. (2011). In vivo precision of the GE Lunar iDXA densitometer for the measurement of total body composition and fat distribution in adults. *European Journal of Clinical Nutrition, 65*, 140–142.

LaForgia, J., Dollman, J., Dale, M.J., Withers, R.T. & Hill, A.M. (2009). Validation of DXA body composition estimates in obese men and women. *Obesity, 17*, 821–826.

Martin, A.D., Spenst, L.F., Drinkwater, D.T. & Clarys, J.P. (1990). Anthropometric estimation of muscle mass in men. *Medicine and Science in Sports and Exercise, 22*, 729–733.

Matiegka, J. (1921). The testing of physical efficiency. *American Journal of Physical Anthropology, 4*, 223–230.

Mitsiopoulos, N., Baumgartner, R.N., Heymsfield, S.B., Lyons, W., Gallagher, D. & Ross R. (1998). Cadaver validation of skeletal muscle measurement by magnetic resonance imaging and computerized tomography. *Journal of Applied Physiology, 85*, 115–122.

Moon, J.R., Eckerson, J.M., Tobkin, S.E., Smith, A.E., Lockwood, C.M., Walter, A.A. et al. (2009). Estimating body fat in NCAA Division I female athletes: a five-compartment model validation of laboratory methods. *European Journal of Applied Physiology, 105*, 119–130.

Peeters, M.W. & Claessens, A.L. (2009). Effect of deviating clothing schemes on the accuracy of body composition measurements by air-displacement plethysmography. *International Journal of Body Composition Research, 7*, 123–129.

Peeters, M.W. & Claessens, A.L. (2010). Effect of different swim caps on the assessment of body volume and percentage body fat by air displacement plethysmography. *Journal of Sports Sciences, 29*, 1–6.

Rössner, S., Bo, W.J., Hiltbrandt, E., Hinson, W., Karstaedt, N., Santago, P. et al. (1990). Adipose tissue determinations in cadavers: a comparison between cross-sectional planimetry and computed tomography. *International Journal of Obesity Research, 14*, 893–902.

Rothney, M.P., Brychta, R.J., Schaefer, E.V., Chen, K.Y. & Skarulis, M.C. (2009). Body composition measured by dual-energy X-ray absorptiometry half-body scans in obese adults. *Obesity, 17*, 1281–1286.

Siri, W.E. (1956). The gross composition of the body. *Advances in Biological and Medical Physics, 4*, 239–280.

Sohlström, A., Wahlund, L.O. & Forsum, E. (1993). Adipose tissue distribution as assessed by magnetic resonance imaging and total body fat by magnetic resonance imaging, underwater weighing, and body-water dilution in healthy women. *American Journal of Nutrition, 58*, 830–838.

Visser, M., Fuerst, T., Lang, T., Salamone, L. & Harris, T.B. (1999). Validity of fan-beam dual-energy X-ray absorptiometry for measuring fat-free mass and leg muscle mass. Health, Aging, and Body Composition Study – Dual-Energy X-ray Absorptiometry and Body Composition Working Group. *Journal of Applied Physiology, 87*, 1513–1520.

Wang, J., Gallagher, D., Thornton, J.C., Yu, W., Horlick, M. & Pi-Sunyer, F.X. (2006). Validation of a 3-dimensional photonic scanner for the measurement of body volumes, dimensions, and percentage body fat. *American Journal of Clinical Nutrition, 83*, 809–816.

Wang, Z.M., Pierson, R.N.Jr. & Heymsfield, S.B. (1992). The five-level model: a new approach to organizing body-composition research. *American Journal of Clinical Nutrition, 56*, 19–28.

Wells, J.C., Treleaven, P. & Cole, T.J. (2007). BMI compared with 3-dimensional body shape: the UK National Sizing Survey. *The American Journal of Clinical Nutrition, 85*, 419–425.

Widdowson, E.M., McCance, R.A. and Spray, C.M. (1951). The chemical composition of the human body, *Clinical Science, 10*, 113–125.

Wilmore, J.H., Vodak, P.A., Parr, R.B., Girandola, R.N. and Billing, J.E. (1980). Further simplification of a method for determination of residual lung volume. *Medicine and Science in Sports and Exercise, 12*, 216–218.

3

PORTABLE METHODS OF BODY COMPOSITION ANALYSIS

Yvonne Mulholland and Catherine Rolland

This chapter will cover:

3.1 Anthropometry
3.2 Near infrared interactance
3.3 Bioelectrical impedance
3.4 Ultrasound

In this chapter field assessment techniques for body composition analysis are considered, in circumstances where access to laboratory equipment is not feasible. There is continued interest in the development of accurate, reproducible and portable methods for analysis, several of which will be outlined in this chapter including anthropometry, near infrared interactance, bioelectrical impedance and ultrasonography.

3.1 Anthropometry

Anthropometry is defined as 'the scientific procedures and processes of acquiring surface anatomical dimensional measurements such as lengths, breadths, girths, and skinfolds of the human body by means of specialist equipment' (Stewart, 2010, p. 455). This enables quantification of absolute dimensions as well as proportions of the human body using portable equipment suitable for field settings. Anthropometric measurements were performed in ancient civilisations and have undergone little change in the last century.

Stature and mass are the most common anthropometric measurements made. Stature can be assessed by a portable stadiometer (a self-standing device with a moveable headboard); an anthropometer (a rod-like device with a moveable right-angled side branch, the long axis of which is held vertically by the measurer); or a

Broca plane (a right-angled headboard which is used in conjunction with a pre-existing vertical surface onto which a measurement is marked). Body mass is assessed by its weight (the force exerted by the product of mass and the earth's gravity), which today is measured almost exclusively by digital scales, which are less prone to calibration errors and damage with movement to different measuring locations than beam balances or spring balances. Assessment of body mass requires a solid floor which is flat. For many other anthropometric measurements, known points on the skin surface, or landmarks, are required. Landmarking is the cornerstone of accurate measuring, and relates surface position to the underlying skeletal structure, or other readily identifiable surface feature. While some bony landmarks are readily identifiable, these still require palpation by a skilled practitioner and, in muscular individuals or those with greater adiposity, they can be very difficult to locate.

Girths require a non-stretch tape which is passed around the body segment and held against the skin surface, or overlying clothing, in circumstances where accessing the skin surface is not feasible. Generally, girths are recorded as maximum girths (e.g. calf girth); minimum girths (e.g. waist or ankle girth), or at a specified point located by landmarking (e.g. chest girth or mid upper-arm girth). In order to be read to acceptable accuracy, tapes should ideally have a stub – a section several centimetres long which is held in one hand, so as not to obscure the zero line where the measurement is taken. Standard technique involves spanning any skin concavities which exist, such as in the lower back at the waist girth.

Measurements of segment length, enabling body proportions to be quantified, include the use of a segmometer, which is essentially a carpenter's tape with moveable side branches, and can measure a point-to-point distance over a curved surface, which avoids the error introduced by measuring at the skin surface. Skeletal breadths are measured by bone calipers or wide-spreading calipers, usually with compression of the overlying soft tissue. Skinfolds, of all anthropometric measurements, are generally the most difficult to acquire and the least accurate. These involve pinching the skin with the thumb and forefinger, pulling it away from its resting position and placing calipers on the fold. The measurement of skinfold thickness, therefore, measures the thickness of a double layer of skin and the underlying subcutaneous adipose tissue. Skinfold sites also require landmarking, as it is well established that a location error in where the fold is measured affects the magnitude of the result.

The sum of skinfolds clearly outperforms body mass index (BMI) as an indicator of adiposity (Sutton, Scott & Reilly, 2009). In addition, the variable fat patterning according to age, ethnicity and level of adiposity means all body regions (i.e. arms, legs and torso) should ideally be included in a skinfold total. The International Society for the Advancement of Kinanthropometry (ISAK) recommends using the sum of eight skinfolds, which, although more time-consuming than approaches using only three or four sites, is likely to be a better indicator of adiposity, and describes fat patterning more effectively. Current protocols developed by ISAK are discussed in more detail in Chapter 7. As with other methods of body composition analysis, the individual being assessed needs to be wearing appropriate clothing, and according to protocols of other measures required, may need to be fasted, voided and recovered from exercise in addition. The skin needs to be dry in order for instruments to be used without slipping, or adhering to areas of the body adjacent to the measurement. For infection control, basic hygiene is essential, and measurements are not made in locations where the skin is broken.

If skinfolds are to be related to total body fatness, then three major assumptions are necessary. First, it is assumed that the skinfold locations measured are representative of all superficial adipose tissue, the thickness of which can be reliably measured by a compressed double fold. Second, it is assumed that subcutaneous adipose tissue represents all fat depots in the body. Third, it is assumed that the person being measured is represented by the sample used to derive the prediction equation and that the reference method (most commonly underwater weighing) is valid.

In all anthropometric methods, technique is important, but especially so in skinfolds. Because adipose tissue is compressible (due to the movement of extracellular fluid, as well as the elastic properties of the tissue itself), the pressure and the time of application of the calipers needs to be standardised. Most calipers have a standard closing pressure (commonly $10\,g.mm^{-2}$) although this does vary between some models. The longer the calipers are applied, the greater the compression and the smaller the reading will be. Protocols for measurement have been developed which seek to record the measurement at the time corresponding to an inflection in the compression curve. Most protocols (including the ISAK protocol) use two seconds to do this, but this is not universal across others, and therefore results are not strictly comparable. Other aspects of technique are also pivotal to reproducible measurements. This centres around having tightly controlled positioning of the person being measured, the measurer, as well as other standardised details which limit the scope for variation and thus error. For illustrative purposes, the ISAK method is described here.

- The site of measurement is located and marked appropriately.
- The measurer's left hand approaches the skin surface from a 90° angle.
- The thumb and forefinger are aligned with the landmark, with the edge of the forefinger of the left hand being directly above the short axis of the landmark.
- The skin is pinched between the forefinger and the thumb, enough (but no more than enough) to generate a parallel sided fold.
- The skinfold is then raised and the calipers are applied exactly 1 cm away from the mark, at a depth corresponding to the midpoint of the fingernail as illustrated in Figure 3.1 (note that this grasp is maintained throughout the measurement).
- The caliper spring tension is released, and the dial is read two seconds afterwards.
- The caliper spring is then depressed, the calipers are removed.
- Finally, the skinfold is released.

This measurement needs to be repeated after the fluid returns to the measurement area (commonly about one minute) and subsequent measurements made, once the measurer is blinded to the first measures. The mean of two or, if these differ by more than 5 per cent from each other, the median of three measurements is used as the skinfold value.

Because of the highly skilled nature of measuring, results can vary widely depending on the observer's experience and the measurement protocol used. An untrained measurer may have a technical error of measurement of 2–3 per cent for stature and 3–4 per cent for girths, and over 15 per cent for skinfolds but with training this technical error or measurement could be dramatically reduced to well below 0.5 per cent for stature and girths and 2.5 per cent for skinfolds. The key message is that although the utility of anthropometric measurements is undermined by large errors,

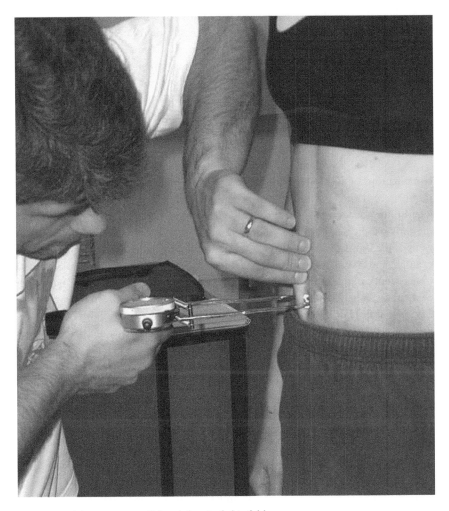

FIGURE 3.1 Measurement of the abdominal skinfold.

these are minimised by detailed adherence to the protocol and thorough and continuous professional training – topics which are considered in Chapters 7 and 10.

In predicting total fatness from anthropometry, it is important to be mindful of the variability of the portion of adipose tissue situated subcutaneously. There is evidence that subcutaneous fat can range from 20 to 70 per cent of total body fat depending on age, sex, ethnicity and degree of fatness (Wagner & Heyward, 1999). This variable partitioning of body fat may present the greatest threat to validity when it comes to selecting a prediction equation for percentage fat. Measurers need to remember that age, ethnicity and level of adiposity all affect fat patterning, underlining the importance of population-specific equations, or those which have undergone separate validation for the groups they are being applied to. It is the great advantage of anthropometry's portability, low cost and straightforward nature that has led many investigators to underestimate the skill required, and limitations of predicting fatness by use of inappropriate equations.

In skilled hands, anthropometry can be a highly reproducible and most useful field method for assessing body composition. It has been suggested that for undernourished patients, skin fold thickness measurements are as useful as more sophisticated methods such as underwater weighing for the estimation of body composition (Probst, Goris, Vandereycken and Van Coppenolle, 2001). This is clearly important because skinfold thickness measurements are more practicable for screening than many other methods, especially for field studies in areas where undernourishment is prevalent.

Of the 100 or more prediction equations available which use various combinations of anthropometric variables, most use different skinfold locations or numbers to define a skinfold total from, and apply different data modelling (e.g. logarithmic, quadratic) to fit the skinfold data to the reference method. Some of the early generalised equations of the 1970s had only fair prediction error (standard error of the estimate ~5 per cent fat, as determined by underwater weighing). If for example a male was measured at 15 per cent fat, then the researcher could only be 67 per cent confident of the actual value falling between 10 per cent and 20 per cent fat, or 95 per cent confident of the actual value falling between 5 per cent and 25 per cent fat. For individual predictions this is an unacceptable level of accuracy, especially in view of the shortcomings of the densitometric method which is generating the dependent variable or reference method. Yet the use of such equations persists in practice for specific athletic or ethnic groups for which they have never been validated. In addition to such validation, prediction equations require a robust method for selecting predictor variables. A study of skinfold equations for estimating body density in youth wrestlers (Stout et al., 1995), highlighted the limited available data for the accuracy of skinfold equations in young populations, suggesting physical activity status may influence which skinfold sites and equations should be used. Another study (Stewart & Hannan, 2000) compared bioelectric impedance analysis (BIA) and anthropometry for predicting fat mass and fat-free mass in 106 male athletes from a wide variety of sports, using DXA as the reference method. The results suggested that skinfold measurements better predicted fat mass (standard error of the estimate 1.7 kg vs. 2.8 kg for skinfolds and BIA respectively) and fat free mass (standard error of the estimate 1.7 kg vs. 2.7 kg respectively) in male athletes than did bioimpedance. This study utilised a stepwise regression method to select the optimal skinfold sites from a selection of 19 locations across the body regions, and concluded that appropriate skinfold selection is a crucial element in the accuracy of a prediction equation for a specific population. Using individual skinfolds, as opposed to a skinfold total, six sites were selected using the entire sample which reduced to two, when a random sub-sample of 82 were used, and validated with the remaining 24 athletes.

$$\text{fat mass (g)} = 331.5(\text{abdominal}) + 356.2(\text{thigh}) + 111.9\text{M} - 9108$$

($R^2 = 0.81$; standard error of the estimate (SEE) $= 1732$ g; $P < 0.001$), where M is body mass in kg; skinfolds in mm.

This raises an important point – that the greater the heterogeneity in a sample, the greater the scope for generalisation of an equation, but the poorer accuracy (i.e. greater the standard error). A balance needs to be struck between having the scope for inference to other groups and a low error. However, a low SEE may still not be effective as a prediction, and it is important to consider total error (TE) in addition.

TE $= [\Sigma(\text{reference method fat mass} - \text{predicted fat mass})^2 / n]$, where n is the number of participants (the same expression is used for FFM). A low TE corresponds to a low y-axis intercept of the prediction regression line, corresponding to a biologically plausible model. The Stewart & Hannan (2000) anthropometric equations for fat mass and FFM have TE of 2.9 per cent and 2.7 per cent respectively. Unfortunately, TE is less widely reported in recent research, limiting easy comparison between predictions.

Further work in anthropometry should continue the validation of existing equations with other groups – especially using more sophisticated multi-compartment models. This will involve the development of more population-specific anthropometric equations in particular for different paediatric, ethnic and specific disease groups. In the meantime, anthropometry remains a useful and reliable method for measuring body composition in the field when performed by an appropriately trained individual to a well-defined protocol.

3.2 Near infrared interactance

Near infrared interactance (NIR) was initially developed as a tool for assessing food composition. It operates on the basis that different types of tissue absorb light at different wavelengths. As pure fat will absorb at 930 nm and pure water at 970 nm, it is possible to obtain percentage body fat and lean tissue mass using prediction equations based on area under the curve of these spectrophotometric parameters (Conway, Norris & Bodwell, 1984). The shape of the interactance spectrum is a function of the amount of fat, water and protein present in the sample. Small portable NIR devices are available to use in nonclinical settings to measure body fat by taking measurements at the biceps site using optical densities from light emissions of 940 and 950 nm (Schreiner, Pitkaniemi, Pekkanen & Salomaa, 1995). When compared to conventional methods of body composition assessment (waist circumference, BMI, waist-to-hip ratio), Schreiner and colleagues demonstrated acceptable reliability of 95.3 per cent and repeatability in trained observers using NIR, on the basis of a lack of significant difference. However, this does not provide evidence of accuracy. Other studies have shown that the NIR device tended to overestimate body fat in lean athletic adults (Brodie & Eston, 1992). Others suggested that NIR tends to underestimate adiposity in fatter individuals and to overestimate it in leaner individuals of both genders (Schreiner et al., 1995). Factors which may also affect percentage body fat predictions include skin colour, variable skin thickness and tissue fluid content. Schreiner and colleagues concluded that until the NIR was able to prove its capability to accommodate for variations in adiposity, age and ethnicity, it provided little advantage in reliability over conventional anthropometric measures of adiposity.

Like skinfolds, NIR measures only subcutaneous adipose tissue and, as a result, it becomes progressively less accurate with individuals who may have substantial visceral fat accumulation. While some factors can be accounted for by the input of descriptive data (stature, mass, frame size, physical activity, age and gender) which inform the prediction model, the validity of such models has still to gain acceptance. However, these input data alone have a large influence on the percentage fat estimation. Justifiable importance is also attributed to the probe placement and reading and therefore training (Schreiner et al., 1995). Like other surrogates for subcutaneous adiposity, there is potential for tissue depth data to be used in their own right, without conversion to percentage fat.

Research by Conway and his group, which based its primary site choice on analysis of NIR at five standard anatomical sites used in skinfold and ultrasound assessment, led to development of a commercial NIR analyser which was designed by the Futrex Corporation (Futrex 5000®, Futrex Corporation, Hagerstown, MD). For measurement a light probe is placed on the participant's biceps brachii. Surprisingly, NIR predictions of fatness from the biceps site alone appear to have smaller prediction errors than those from multiple sites – possibly due to less potential for noise introduced by other anatomical structures. The NIR light enters the tissues to a depth of 4 cm and is reflected back to a detector which measures the optical density at set wavelengths (940 and 950 nm). Based on the principle that optical density is linearly and inversely proportional to percentage body fat, the smaller the optical density, the greater the fat content.

Although these measurements appear to be repeatable, it has been claimed that Futrex consistently underestimates percentage body fat (Wagner & Heyward, 1999), and the error is greater with increasing body fat. In light of the possibility of large errors, and the lack of widespread acceptance in the scientific community, the use of Futrex 5000® and smaller version Futrex 1000® are not generally recommended for assessing percentage fat, because the prediction errors are unacceptably high.

Despite this general finding amongst research, some studies reported a contrary view at similar times to these recommendations. One study assessed percentage body fat in athletic individuals (Fornetti, Pivarnik, Foley & Fiechter, 1999) and examined the validity of NIR (using the Futrex 5000® biceps measurement) and BIA in young female athletes in comparison to DXA. Both BIA and NIR were shown to be valid, reliable and, when converted to percentage body fat, they demonstrated low predictive error of ~1.8 per cent. This demonstrated the potential of the instrument in particular populations, but did suggest that measurement instruments require revised algorithms, which is consistent with evidence athletes may have different fat patterning from non-athletic individuals.

Another study used NIR to investigate variable factors influencing fat patterning such as including level of obesity and ethnicity, in predicting fatness assessed by DXA (Jennings et al., 2010). In this study, despite a significant relationship in prediction of body fat between DXA and NIR, it demonstrated an under-prediction using a newer Futrex-6100® model single site NIR in black women and also obese black women. The error also increased with increasing adiposity, and further demonstrated the population specificity of measurements. In particular populations, light absorption variability due to increased melanin may need to be included in the NIR algorithms. Differences in peripheral and visceral adiposity may also have to be included in predictive alterations. At present, in the morbidly obese, NIR may not prove an accurate tool for measurement.

In a more recent publication, as part of the Finrisk92 study, obese individuals were assessed for a number of parameters including BMI, waist-to-hip ratio (WHR), waist circumference and body fat as assessed by NIR. Once again the Futrex 5000® was used for measurements of biceps. These were used to predict cardiovascular disease (CVD), coronary heart disease and ischaemic stroke risk in a large mixed-gender population study. In this population whilst NIR was a significant predictor of CVD risk, it was no better than other measures of obesity, including BMI, waist circumference (WC) and WHR, in terms of predictive power of risk. Also, for ischaemic stroke it was a poorer predictor than the other currently popular methods of BMI, WC and WHR. Thus, overall NIR was deemed no better than BMI or WHR (Pajunen et al., 2011).

Although field-based methods are required to assess fatness in larger scale studies, and some studies suggest NIR may be a useful and valid tool, the balance of available data suggest instrument reliability is somewhat variable. Development and benchmarking of revised models together with improved algorithms for predicting fatness in different groups which offer better predictability and reliability is required before the technique gains wider acceptance.

3.3 Bioelectrical impedance

Bioelectrical impedance analysis (BIA) is currently the only field technique with the capability of predicting total body water (TBW) and, indirectly, fat-free mass (FFM). The ability of body tissues to conduct an electrical current has been recognised for over a hundred years (Ellis, 2000). Bioelectrical impedance utilises this principle and enables the measurement of conductivity of a small alternating electrical current through the body tissues. Water, due to its electrolyte rich content, will easily conduct electrical currents in comparison to fat, which is a poor conductor, as a result of its anhydrous nature. In BIA, electrodes are placed on the body and a small current introduced. A voltage drop occurs between two electrodes when there is opposition to the flow of current and its path through the body exploits these differences in conductivity of fat and water. Impedance, as determined by this voltage drop is therefore inversely related to conductance. Impedance (Z) has two contributing factors: reactance (Xc) and resistance (R), where

$$Z^2 = R^2 + Xc^2$$

Resistance is the restriction of current flow and is inversely proportional to fluid volumes and, assuming constant hydration, to fat-free mass in addition. Ohm's law states that the current between two points varies according to the voltage, and is inversely proportional to the resistance. Resistance is proportional to the specific resistivity and length of a material but is inversely related to cross-sectional area (Deurenberg-Yap & Deurenberg, 2001; Kyle et al., 2004). Therefore resistance, in a uniform material, can be defined as proportional to length and cross sectional area by the equation:

$$R = Pl / A$$

and also

$$R = pL^2 / V$$

where p is resistivity of the material at a given temperature, A is area, L is length and where A x L =V, volume. (Kyle et al., 2004; Wagner & Heyward, 1999).

Reactance is the term used to take account of the capacitance of cell membranes and tissue interfaces. A capacitor has the ability to store energy and consists of two conducting surfaces separated by an insulating substance. In this case, the cell membrane consists of non-conducting lipid and permeable protein ion channels, which separate the intra- and extracellular fluids creating an electrical gradient. Reactance helps us determine intracellular fluid volumes by current dependent methods because capacitance decreases with increased current frequency. A third term, which is still to be accurately defined, is the phase angle. Reactance results in a displacement or 'lag' of the current behind the voltage. The phase angle represents, in degrees, the voltage lead over current and is the arc-tangent of the ratio of reactance over resistance. The relationship shows that the higher the degree, the better the cell membrane integrity, thus, reactance. The phase angle thus examines the linear relationship between vectors of tissue hydration (resistance) and cell membrane integrity (reactance). It is being used in diseased states to quantify nutritional status and as a prognostic indicator in chronic disease states although the lack of reference values is recognised as a limitation.

The BIA method relies on prediction equations to calculate TBW and FFM. These are not only population- specific, but are based on a number of assumptions. Calculations for TBW and FFM are based on the impedance calculation that body volume is equal to height^2/resistance. The underlying equations that derive this relationship are based on the principle that, as stated above, in an isotropic and cylindrical material resistance is proportional to conductor length and inversely proportional to cross-sectional area. What is seldom acknowledged, however, is that height is not actually the conductor length but rather the wrist to ankle distance in tetra–polar arrangements. Cross-sectional area also varies by position because the body is not uniformly cylindrical and, in addition, tissue conductivity, far from being constant, varies considerably between different tissues. It is recognised that although the trunk contains a large proportion of total body water, because of its large cross-sectional area, it represents only a small percentage of the total resistance which is converse to the limbs, despite their smaller area (Wagner & Heyward, 1999). This is exploited in the more recently introduced segmental BIA analysis which independently assesses body segments. The other assumption made in BIA is that the reactance component of impedance is negligible (while impedance is overwhelmingly dominated by resistance, reactance can be ~1 per cent of impedance at 50 KHz) but this is not the case as shown in multifrequency BIA (MF-BIA), where higher frequencies are required to traverse the cell membrane (Earthman, Traughber, Dobratz & Howell, 2007; Ellis, 2001).

A number of electrode arrangements can be utilised in BIA measurement but the standard technique is the tetrapolar instrument where paired electrodes are placed, most frequently on the right side of the body, and measurements taken along the longitudinal axes of the body. With the participant lying supine on a non-conducting surface with limbs partially abducted, electrodes are placed on the dorsum of the hand and foot, near the metacarpo-phalangeal and metatarso-phalangeal joints. Further electrodes are placed between the distal prominences of the radius and ulna and also the midpoint between the lateral and medial ankle malleoli (Lukaski, 1987). More recently, bipolar and octapolar arrangements have become common and, thus, there are now many variations of this technique. Bipedal instruments have been developed which appear similar to bathroom scales and have integrated metal electrode plates on which to stand and simultaneously measure bioimpedance and weight. As such, no conductivity information is derived from the arms or torso.

Regardless of the electrode arrangement used, most commercially available models are based on a single frequency current of 50kHz, which represents a critical frequency in which current theoretically passes into both extra and intracellular fluids. Stahn and colleagues (2007) argue, however, that the standard 50kHz is not sufficiently high to penetrate the cellular membrane fully, and thus measurements at this frequency are more influenced by extracellular than intracellular fluid. A weak current is transmitted at this low current from the outer electrodes and voltage drop is measured by the inner electrodes. With the use of predictive equations, estimates of total body water are determined from these measurements, combined with age, stature, mass and gender data. These predictions have utility in healthy, euhydrated individuals represented by the prediction sample population (in terms of age, gender and ethnicity). However, they fail to allow for fluctuation in total body water.

More recently MF-BIA instruments have been developed where a range of low to high frequencies is utilised. Overall, the principles of MF-BIA are to allow measurement of both extracellular and intracellular fluid compartments.

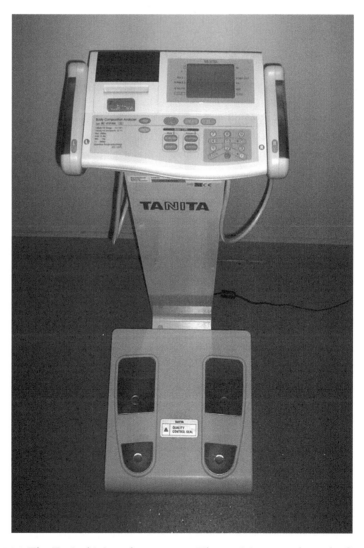

FIGURE 3.2 The Tanita bioimpedance system. The participant stands on the footplate, clasps the handles, and raises these laterally for the measurement.

Theoretically, low frequencies are unable to be conducted across the cell membrane due to its capacitance arising largely from the lipid component. Thus, at low frequencies, measurements will calculate the extracellular fluid compartments. In contrast, at high frequencies, reactance of the cell membrane decreases and therefore the current should pass through the cell membrane allowing assessment of intracellular water and thus TBW.

Further developments from this have also led to the introduction of bio-impedance spectroscopy (BIS) where, as the name suggests, a more complex model over a spectrum of frequencies (5–1000 kHz) is used. This allows examination of body segments, or breakdown of the body into a number of cylinders, which is a logical development because impedance is proportionally greater in the limbs (Heymsfield, Wang, Baumgartner & Ross, 1997). Its advantages are that it is less influenced by disease states, which alter body hydration status and impact on results of single-frequency (SF-BIA) and MF-BIA. Prediction models for BIS, (also in MF-BIA), are used to estimate the optimal frequencies for measurement of intra- and extracellular fluid.

Prediction equations for FFM are based on an assumed constant hydration status (~73 per cent in adults) and thus are influenced by a number of situations in which the normal body water distribution is altered. Body fat percentage can be calculated by deriving FFM from TBW and deriving fat mass by subtraction from total mass. Individual assessment, if not using a specific prediction model, can therefore be inaccurate not only by assumption errors of hydration, but by precision and rounding errors arising from mass measurement. Results can be affected due to alterations in fluids by factors including food consumption and exercise. Impedance measurements may be reduced up to four hours post-ingestion, thus measurements eight hours post-ingestion are optimal (Deurenberg, Weststrate, Paymans & van der Kooy 1988). Exercise can also affect tissue perfusion with increased blood flow resulting in reduced resistance. Insensible losses from excessive sweating will, however, result in increased resistivity due to loss of body water. Again, it is suggested that several hours must pass before BIA analysis can be performed post-exertion. Any variable affecting hydration status, and thus, the balance of intra and extracellular fluids, can become a confounding variable. Participants are asked to void the bladder before measurements can be taken. Alcohol consumption, diuretic medications and caffeine will dehydrate and specific disease states can result in compartmental fluid shifts. Particular patient groups affected include those with heart, renal or liver failure where fluid shifts can be substantial. Research in patient groups where hydration status can be altered is of increasing interest in long-term monitoring of nutritional status and may offer a clinical tool in assessing long-term body composition changes. Orthostatic changes may also influence BIA readings due to changes in extracellular fluid and thus postural position may also influence the impedance in the limbs. Other factors which influence impedance values are in disease states where there can be altered tissue perfusion, muscular wasting, variability in limb proportions, amputations and variations in skin temperature (Kushner, Gudivaka & Schoeller, 1996).

On the whole, BIA's advantages centre on its relative affordability compared to alternative methods for body composition analysis in the clinical setting, together with the lack of clothing changes required for measuring. These enable patients with mobility and body image issues, which would normally exclude them from other forms of body composition measurements, to be measured. For the technician, BIA requires minimal training and gives highly reproducible results. It is also portable, non-invasive and safe for participant evaluation. However, BIA's disadvantages include the regular calibration of instruments required to obtain reproducible and reliable results. A calibration system has yet to be developed that would provide a standard against the range of human values, particularly in ethnic groups (Houtkooper, Lohman, Going & Howell, 1996). Standardisation of electrode placement may also increase the accuracy of predictions. Another difficulty arises using prediction equations and linear regression analysis from a specific population in that they cannot be extrapolated for widespread clinical use. Particular populations where this may be apparent include those near the extremes of body weight, morphological variations and athletic individuals. Practical difficulties can also occur, depending on the population in question, if there are mobility issues or difficulties which prevent patients lying comfortably or standing for prolonged periods during measurements. Segmental analyses may also provide more practical methods of prediction in these groups.

One recent study (Rush, Cowley, Freitas & Luke, 2006) examined the validity of hand to foot bioimpedance measurements in subjects in lying or standing position. In this study of 205 volunteers aged 6–89 years, they demonstrated that supine impedance was consistently higher than that acquired standing. Changes in resistance were also measured every 30 seconds over an 11-minute period and showed that resistance over time is reduced with standing but increases with lying. Although there were no gender differences they examined resistance against age and found that changes in resistance over time reduced with increasing age, possibly correlating to age-related changes in vascular tone. From their study they were able to tabulate adjustments required for each age sector. This may provide a practical method for field assessment in patients with poorer mobility if population-specific criteria are utilised.

Another recent study (Moon et al., 2008) examined both laboratory and field assessment methods for calculation of percentage body fat compared to validated laboratory multiple compartment models (in this study the Siri three-compartment model). As discussed in Chapter 2, multi-compartment models are the best predictors of body fat, but they are impractical for routine use. In this study, using a population-specific equation, BIA was shown to have an acceptable total error value unlike other field assessment instruments, NIR and circumference-based military equations. Their study supported the use of BIA in Caucasian men when neither air displacement plethysmography (ADP) nor densitometry is feasible. Unlike many previous studies which have failed to show any significant agreement between a multicomponent model and the specific BIA model, this gives further support to BIA being a comparative practical field-based instrument. However, they did also note that as a single frequency, it cannot detect changes in intracellular fluid.

More innovative work has recently been undertaken in BIA assessment of skeletal mass which is useful in assessing malnutrition, catabolic states and sarcopenia, the loss of muscle mass with ageing. Initial studies have examined the skeletal muscle mass in the lower body at fixed standard frequencies (Salinari et al., 2003). A more recent study has used models to assess muscle volume in upper and lower limbs with MF tetrapolar BIA in young males. They compared the results against a model derived from magnetic resonance imaging (MRI). Using a new mathematical approach, which was not reliant on a sample specific population (Stahn, Terblanche & Strobel, 2007), muscle volume estimates in both arm and leg were not different from those measured using MRI. Multiple BIA measurements were shown to be more accurate in measuring lower limb volume as shown by a reduced SEE at 500 kHz as opposed to the upper limb where frequency alterations did not improve accuracy. They concluded that multiple frequency analysis may improve estimates of muscle-mass volumes of lower limbs in healthy males. (Stahn et al., 2007). Elsewhere, however, MF-BIS has been used in estimating arm muscle mass, using a model to estimate total muscle mass, against MRI and total body potassium with promising results. This may provide an alternative, easy and practical measurement for estimating total muscle mass in specific settings (Carter et al., 2009).

Bioimpedance is now also being investigated as a non-invasive tool for monitoring fluid status in heart failure patients providing more information on an outpatient basis regarding fluid overload and potentially preventing unnecessary hospital admission. Its use may, however, be limited in patients with significant peripheral oedema (Tanino et al., 2009). More recently BIA has been adopted to detect myocardial ischaemia, and also in renal patients who are also at a high risk of fluid overload and hypertension, both of which are poor prognostic indicators, and further research is warranted with these groups. Overall, the use of BIA techniques continues to expand. It is proving to be an inexpensive, portable tool in field assessment of not only FFM but in predicting TBW, defining extra and intracellular components and also in estimates of muscle mass itself. It is becoming a useful clinical tool in assessing chronic disease prognosis by use of phase angle although optimal cut-offs for prognostic indication is required. Its use in outpatient monitoring of conditions where fluid overload leads to significant morbidity and mortality is also to be further evaluated. Studies in the field of prosthetic engineering are in their preliminary stages but BIA assessment again may provide a useful tool in investigating composition in amputees and disabled sports athletes. Further research which provides composition models which are appropriate for the extremes of body composition such as athletes, eating disordered or obese patients, and also in children is required. Compliance with the necessary prerequisites for BIA measurement validity can be problematic, and increasing rigour in future studies will be required to address this.

3.4 Ultrasound

Since the 1950s ultrasound technology has become a crucial and versatile diagnostic instrument within the medical field. The innovative use of ultrasound technology specifically for measurement of body composition was, however, initially explored in agricultural research. Measurements of adiposity on animal carcasses produced essential data which were later extrapolated to human studies (Stouffer, 1968) in aerospace research who examined its use in determining fat, muscle, bone and tissue volumes. Since then, ultrasound technology has become increasingly portable and therefore potentially offers a practical field technique for measurement of adipose tissue depth and prediction of adiposity.

Today there are a number of ultrasound devices available, but until recently their size precluded easy use in the field. Ultrasound scanners are all based on the same fundamental principles. Sound comprises mechanical waves generated from the disturbance of particles in a medium. Its main characteristics are therefore frequency, wavelength, velocity and amplitude. Ultrasound frequencies are classified as greater than 2 kHz. At these frequencies, beyond the sensitivity of human hearing, ultrasound technology utilises sound waves to identify materials of varying density and generate images. In practical clinical and research fields higher frequencies of 1–10 MHz are generally utilised. Each device has a transducer comprised of piezoelectric crystals which transform electrical energy into pulsed sound waves. To permit transduction of the sound waves through tissue, a water-soluble gel is required as a medium, preventing air entry (which would result in an artefact). In assessment of body adipose tissue the sound waves are transmitted longitudinally through the skin and are echoed back from tissue interfaces, in this case the adipose tissue-muscle interface. These interfaces are detected in tissues due to differences in 'acoustic impedance', a term in ultrasound research which expresses speed of sound through the material in relation to its density. (Note: this differs from electrical impedance as described in Section 3.3.) The velocity of sound waves through a material is dependent on its density. The higher the impedance the more the waves will be reflected rather than transmitted. Ultrasound has been shown to be capable of detecting tissue density interfaces to 1 mm precision (Fanelli & Kuczmarski, 1984). The reflected waves are detected by the transducer and converted back to an electrical signal which can then be transformed into an image. The processor calculates tissue depth from multiplication of velocity of the sound wave and time interval between sound wave emission and returning echo (distance = (speed × time / 2) as time includes pulse travelling to and echoing back from tissues). This describes 'A-mode' imaging, amplitude modulation, where one-dimensional information of the distance between the single line from transducer and reflector is provided. A-mode imaging is the simplest form of ultrasound and detects differences in amplitude of reflections to give an impression of depth. Amplitudes will vary between tissues depending on their impedance. Reflected waves at each tissue interface can be assessed as spikes on a time-amplitude plot.

Alternatively, a two-dimensional image by way of 'B-mode', or brightness modulation, ultrasonography can be generated. In this form of ultrasound an array of transducers scan to produce multiple echoes which are graded in a traditional grey scale image (Starck, Dietz & Piersma, 2001). In contrast to the spikes produced in A-mode imaging, B-mode converts the echoes into dots where the brightness reflects the amplitude of the reflected signal. Thus a large amplitude signal produces a bright dot of near-white and a low amplitude signal produces a near-black dot. An ultrasound pulse sent through the varying tissues can therefore produce an image from the spectrum of bright spots reflected from the underlying structures at their interfaces. Other modalities of ultrasound include 'M-mode' imaging (which conveys movement information), and Doppler ultrasound, (where the reflected echo frequencies vary according to speed and direction of the reflector – for instance in arterial or venous blood flow). Three-dimensional ultrasound scanners are also now available and are being developed for portable applications.

Ultrasound has many advantages in field research of body composition. Low-weight portable machines have now been developed which make its use practical for field-based measurements and thus transferable to both research and clinical settings where estimations of adiposity are required. It has an advantage over many other medical imaging techniques as it does not involve radiation, has negligible risk, is non-invasive and painless for the participant.

Recently it has been recognised that it has the potential to replace skinfold thickness measurements; however, it is important to remember that ultrasound measurements are not directly equivalent to skinfolds: they comprise a single uncompressed adipose tissue layer plus skin, whereas a skinfold is a compressed double layer of adipose tissue and skin. However, skinfold thickness can be difficult to determine by calipers in some individuals for a number of reasons including the need for palpation, alterations in compression of tissue due to age and hydration status, and adherence of adipose tissue to the underlying muscle fascia. In the obese patient, the skinfold can be difficult to raise with parallel sides and the calipers may slip or have an aperture insufficiently wide to measure the grasp (Kuczmarski, Fanelli & Koch, 1987). Under such circumstances, ultrasound offers more versatility and comparative studies of both techniques have supported its effectiveness in predicting body density (Fanelli & Kuczmarski, 1984). However, reliability can also be variable given that results are very much contingent on operator skill. Further work (Kuczmarski et al., 1987) assessed the comparability of ultrasound and calipers and demonstrated significant correlation between both measures across all sites, in particular triceps, biceps and thigh. This study noted ultrasound measures at the biceps, subscapular, waist and thigh to correlate better than caliper measurements with against body density. However, as was highlighted in Chapter 2, the densitometric method is no longer considered the criterion it was in previous decades, so this finding needs to be interpreted with caution.

No technique is without its imperfections, however, and the main disadvantages of ultrasound include its cost and training requirements. Regarding the preferred portable technique there are a number of contradictory studies and this may be influenced by the weight differences in participants. Many of the studies have failed to show reproducible models or techniques that may be extrapolated within the population to all individuals regardless of body mass. The technique in ultrasound measurement is crucially important because inadequate training may result in multiple echoes and inconsistent results, secondary to operator errors such as incorrect positioning of the transducer and tissue compression. The correct probe position is perpendicular to the surface as illustrated in Figure 3.3; however,

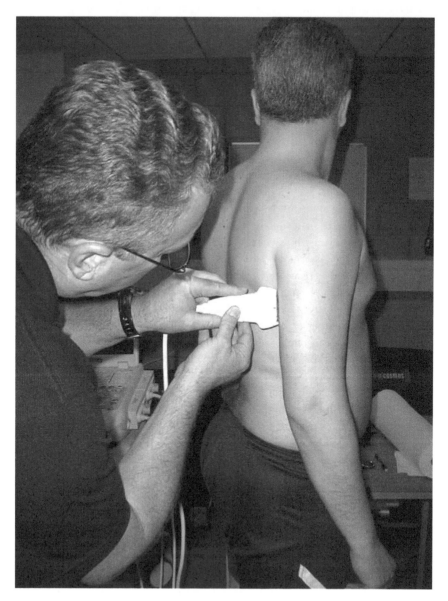

FIGURE 3.3 A portable ultrasound scanner measurement of the upper arm.

deviation from this can result in attenuation of the signal. Perpendicular placement allows optimal tissue reflection to assess depth which, if not correctly positioned, may otherwise be overestimated due to refraction error.

It is also important to consider the frequencies used. Wavelength, the distance travelled by sound in one cycle, is important in achieving a good quality resolution. This is inversely balanced with frequency as:

$$\text{Wavelength} = \text{velocity} / \text{frequency}$$

therefore a high frequency results in poorer penetration (Starck et al., 2001). Higher frequency is useful in superficial structures whereas lower frequency better analyses deeper structures (Jacobson, 2007). For quantifying adipose tissue a flat transducer is recommended, with frequencies of 7–10 MHz for typical participants, and higher frequencies for leaner, and lower frequencies for fatter individuals respectively.

In more recent studies portable ultrasound has been used to determine percentage body fat. In one such study (Pineau, Guihard-Costa & Bocquet, 2007) ultrasound was compared with BIA and ADP against reference measurements from DXA in 89 sedentary subjects aged 18–60 years. All techniques correlated with DXA results but ultrasound produced the highest correlation in both genders, and lower total error. (The results of ADP and BIA demonstrated significant levels of bias.) If we accept DXA as a valid reference method, these results suggest that ultrasound has a higher accuracy and reliability than BIA or ADP.

A further study by the same group looked at the validity of A-mode ultrasound against DXA in 93 male and female athletes, demonstrating high correlation and low total error. A similar prediction model for estimates of total body fat was used and this proved accurate in this particular sample of athletes from a narrow BMI range, contrasting significantly from the previous sample of hospital patients with a wider BMI variation (Pineau, Fillard & Bocquet, 2009). Another study has attempted to develop an accurate equation for prediction of body density of sumo wrestlers (Saito et al., 2003). In this study, B-mode ultrasound was utilised to measure subcutaneous thickness at nine body sites alongside circumference measurements and BIA. Body density was also measured using underwater weighing in 24 wrestlers and 24 age- and weight-matched individuals. In these groups, simple linear and multiple regression analysis helped to identify the measurements to derive predictive equations for body density. Their overall conclusions were, however, that this equation was only valid in sumo wrestlers and could not be extrapolated to other normal or overweight athletes.

Another role of ultrasound is assessment of intra-abdominal adipose tissue which has had a long reported history as a marker of increased cardiovascular risk. The techniques of CT and MRI, as outlined in Chapter 2, are currently more accepted for assessing visceral fat but their availability and practicalities of measurement are limited by equipment size, cost and radiation exposure. Whilst waist circumference measurements may offer a tool to estimate central adiposity, ultrasound was assessed for its validity in 19 obese subjects against CT, MRI and anthropometry. Using specific criteria for ultrasound measurement analysis they demonstrated a significant correlation (0.81, p<0.001) between single slice CT (cross sectional scan, cm², at the level of the lumbar vertebrae L4–5) and ultrasound (measured at the posterior edge of abdominal muscles to lumbar spine) independent of which sonographer acquired the measurements. Similar results were obtained on repeat assessments three months later after weight loss in the same individuals. They also demonstrated a high correlation with waist circumference. To assess reproducibility the mean of main distances was used and these distances were assessed in two ultrasonographers. The significant correlation between data from each was 0.94 which demonstrates good reproducibility, the absence of which has often been a criticism in other similar studies (Stolk et al., 2001). However, the cross-sectional adipose tissue area of a single slice does not necessarily reflect the total volume of adipose tissue and this distinction is often overlooked in similar studies.

In follow up to this work this group further assessed intra-abdominal fat (IAF) in 600 patients at high risk of vessel disease in the SMART study (Secondary Manifestations of Arterial Disease – Stolk et al., 2003). Ultrasound measurements of intra-abdominal fat along with waist measurements were used to predict metabolic syndrome risk factors. The correlation coefficients for IAF as measured by ultrasound showed a significantly higher association with cardiovascular metabolic risk factors such as glucose, total cholesterol, high density lipoprotein, cholesterol, triacylglycerol, than did waist measurement. This may not be surprising, as waist is not a direct measurement of fatness combining subcutaneous and visceral depots using an assumed circular model. Crucially, subcutaneous fat measured by ultrasound did not correlate with the same metabolic variables. Thus, the utility of ultrasound rests on its ability to assess the more health-harming depots, as well as being an alternative to assessing subcutaneous fat, for instance on overweight individuals where skinfolds may be difficult to raise.

Ultrasound, under strict protocols, may provide a simple, reliable estimate of IAF, as compared with the more expensive and less readily available CT and MRI, and also DXA which is becoming a more widely accepted reference technique for body fat estimation (Pineau et al., 2007). Overall, the limited research in this field is somewhat surprising, considering its safety, utility and cost advantages. As a tool it is inexpensive and portable but evidence is lacking concerning its reproducibility and no single model has yet been validated for standard use in all individuals. Such research would establish representative sites, and reduce the number of unnecessary readings. Computerised sampling approaches to images may enhance the accuracy of ultrasound measurements in the future. Development of a standardised procedure of measuring adipose tissue thickness – for instance, in relation to the pressure applied to the probe for measurement, will enable inter-laboratory comparisons to be more valid. Ultrasound is likely to play a pivotal role in the quantification of tissue compressibility during skinfold measurement, which may vary within and between individuals. In addition, developments which quantify central adiposity accurately and effectively may also inform the design of new equipment in both research and clinical settings.

Portable techniques offer a considerable advantage for use in field or clinical settings where laboratory facilities are unavailable. However, in the wealth of literature including such techniques, some of the science remains poor. Many of the purported validations of such portable methods rely on criterion methods which are no longer considered acceptable. Others quote high correlation, in terms of relationship, without reporting agreement. In spite of this, without recourse to conversion into percentage fat, these raw data represent valuable surrogates for body composition. While standardisation and training criteria are well established for anthropometry, they have yet to be universally accepted. For other techniques, developing a training and quality assurance infrastructure to enable inter-laboratory standardisation remains a priority.

References

Brodie, D.A. & Eston, R.G. (1992). Body fat estimations by electrical impedance and infra-red interactance. *International Journal of Sports Medicine, 13*, 319–325.

Carter, M., Zhu, F., Kotanko, P., Kuhlmann, M., Ramirez, L., Heymsfield, S.B. et al. (2009). Assessment of body composition in dialysis patients by arm bioimpedance compared to MRI and ^{40}K measurements. *Blood Purification, 27*, 330–337.

Conway, J.M., Norris, K.H. & Bodwell, C.E. (1984). A new approach for the estimation of body composition: infrared interactance. *American Journal of Clinical Nutrition, 40*, 1123–1130.

Deurenberg, P., Weststrate, J.A., Paymans, I. & van der Kooy, K. (1988). Factors affecting bioelectrical impedance measurements in humans. *European Journal of Clinical Nutrition, 42*, 1017–1022.

Deurenberg-Yap, M. & Deurenberg, P. (2001) Bioelectrical impedance: from theories to applications. *Malaysian Journal of Nutrition, 7*, 67–74.

Earthman, C., Traughber, D., Dobratz, J. & Howell, W. (2007). Bioimpedance spectroscopy for clinical assessment of fluid distribution and body cell mass. *Nutrition in Clinical Practice, 22*, 389–405.

Ellis, K.J. (2000). Human body composition: *in vivo* methods. *Physiological Reviews, 80*, 649–680.

Ellis, K.J. (2001). Selected body composition methods can be used in field studies. *The Journal of Nutrition, 131*, 1589S–1595S.

Fanelli, M.T. & Kuczmarski, R.J. (1984). Ultrasound as an approach to assessing body composition. *American Journal of Clinical Nutrition, 39*, 703–709.

Fornetti, W.C., Pivarnik, J.M., Foley, J.M. & Fiechter, J.J. (1999). Reliability and validity of body composition measures in female athletes. *Journal of Applied Physiology, 87*, 1114–1122.

Heymsfield, S.B., Wang, Z., Baumgartner, R.N. & Ross, R. (1997). Human body composition: advances in models and methods. *Annual Review of Nutrition, 17*, 527–558.

Houtkooper, L.B., Lohman, T.G., Going, S.B. & Howell, W.H. (1996). Why bioelectrical impedance analysis should be used for estimating adiposity. *American Journal of Clinical Nutrition, 64*, 436S–448S.

Jacobson, J.A. (2007). *Fundamentals of Musculoskeletal Ultrasound*. Philadelphia, PA: Saunders Elsevier.

Jennings, C.J., Micklesfield, L.K., Lambert, M.I., Lambert, E.V., Collins, M. & Goedecke, J.H. (2010). Comparison of body fatness measurements by near infra-red reactance and dual-energy X-ray absorptiometry in normal-weight and obese black and white women. *British Journal of Nutrition, 103*, 1065–1069.

Kuczmarski, R.J., Fanelli, M.T. & Koch, G.G. (1987). Ultrasonic assessment of body composition in obese adults: overcoming the limitations of the skinfold caliper. *American Journal of Clinical Nutrition, 45*, 717–724.

Kushner, R.F., Gudivaka, R. & Schoeller, D.A. (1996). Clinical characteristics influencing bioelectrical impedance analysis measurements. *American Journal of Clinical Nutrition, 64*, 423S–427S.

Kyle, U.G., Bosaeus, I., De Lorenzo, A.D., Deurenberg, P., Elia, M., Gomez, J.M. & Composition of the ESPEN Working Group (2004). Bioelectrical impedance analysis – Part I: Review of principles and methods. *Clinical Nutrition, 23*, 1226–1243.

Lukaski, H.C. (1987). Methods for the assessment of human body composition: traditional and new. *American Journal of Clinical Nutrition, 46*, 537–556.

Moon, J.R., Tobkin, S.E., Smith, A.E., Roberts, M.D., Ryan, E.D., Dalbo, V.J. et al. (2008). Percent body fat estimations in college men using field and laboratory methods: a three-compartment model approach. *Dynamic Medicine, 7*, published online: doi:10.1186/1476-5918-7-7.

Pajunen, P., Jousilahti, P., Borodulin, K., Harald, K., Tuomilehto, J. & Salomaa, V. (2011). Body fat measured by a near-infrared interactance device as a predictor of cardiovascular events: The FINRISK'92 cohort. *Obesity, 19*, 848–852.

Pineau, J.-C., Fillard, J.R. & Bocquet, N. (2009). Ultrasound techniques applied to body fat measurement in male and female athletes. *Journal of Athletic Training, 44*, 142–147.

Pineau, J.-C., Guihard-Costa, A.M. & Bocquet, M. (2007). Validation of ultrasound techniques applied to body fat measurement. A comparison between ultrasound techniques, air displacement plethysmography and bioelectrical impedance vs. dual-energy X-ray absorptiometry. *Annals of Nutrition and Metabolism, 51*, 421–427.

Probst, M., Goris, M., Vandereycken, W. & Van Coppenolle, H. (2001). Body composition of anorexia nervosa patients assessed by underwater weighing and skinfold-thickness measurements before and after weight gain. *American Journal of Clinical Nutrition, 73*, 190–197.

Rush, E.C., Crowley, J., Freitas, I.F. & Luke, A. (2006). Validity of hand-to-foot measurement of bioimpedance: Standing compared with lying position. *Obesity, 14*, 252–257.

Saito, K., Nakaji, S., Umeda, T., Shimoyama, T., Sugawara, K. & Yamamoto, Y. (2003). Development of predictive equations for body density of sumo wrestlers using B-mode ultrasound for the determination of subcutaneous fat thickness. *British Journal of Sports Medicine, 37*, 144–148.

Salinari, S., Bertuzzi, A., Mingrone, G., Capristo, E., Scarfone, A. & Greco, A.V. (2003). Bioimpedance analysis: a useful technique for assessing appendicular lean soft tissue mass and distribution. *Journal of Applied Physiology, 94*, 1552–1556.

Schreiner, P.J., Pitkaniemi, J., Pekkanen, J. & Salomaa, V.V. (1995). Reliability of near-infrared interactance body fat assessment relative to standard anthropometric techniques. *Journal of Clinical Epidemiology, 48*, 1361–1367.

Stahn, A., Terblanche, E. & Strobel, G. (2007). Modeling upper and lower limb muscle volume by bioelectrical impedance analysis. *Journal of Applied Physiology, 103,* 1428–1435.

Starck, J.M., Dietz, M.W. & Piersma, T. (2001). The assessment of body composition and other parameters by ultrasound scanning, body composition analysis of animals. In J.R. Speakman (Ed.) *Body Composition Analysis of Animals: A Handbook of Non-Destructive Methods* (pp. 188–210). Cambridge: Cambridge University Press.

Stewart, A.D. (2010). Kinanthropometry and body composition: a natural home for 3D photonic scanning. *Journal of Sports Sciences, 28,* 455–457.

Stewart, A.D. & Hannan, W.J. (2000). Prediction of fat and fat-free mass in male athletes using dual X-ray absorptiometry as the reference method. *Journal of Sports Sciences, 18,* 263–274.

Stolk, R.P., Meijer, R., Mali, W.P., Grobbee, D.E., van der Graaf, Y. & Secondary Manifestations of Arterial Disease Study Group (2003). Ultrasound measurements of intraabdominal fat estimate the metabolic syndrome better than do measurements of waist circumference. *American Journal of Clinical Nutrition, 77,* 857–860.

Stolk, R.P., Wink, O., Zelissen, P.M., Meijer, R., van Gils, A.P. & Grobbee, D.E. (2001). Validity and reproducibility of ultrasonography for the measurement of intra-abdominal adipose tissue. *International Journal of Obesity and Related Metabolic Disorders, 25,* 1346–1351.

Stouffer, J.R. (1968). *Ultrasonic Determination of Body Composition* (No. AMRL-TR-68-61). Wright-Patterson Air Force Base, OH: Aerospace Medical Research Laboratory.

Stout, J.R., Housh, T.J., Johnson, G.O., Housh, D.J., Evans, S.A. & Eckerson, J.M. (1995). Validity of skinfold equations for estimating body density in youth wrestlers. *Medicine and Science in Sports and Exercise, 27,* 1321–1325.

Sutton, L., Scott, M. & Reilly, T. (2009). A comparison of laboratory-based and field-based methods of body composition analysis. In P.A. Hume & A.D. Stewart (Eds.) *Kinanthropometry XI: 2008 Pre-Olympic Congress Anthropometry Research* (pp. 8–14). Auckland: International Society for the Advancement of Kinanthropometry.

Tanino, Y., Shite, J., Paredes, O.L., Shinke, T., Ogasawara, D., Sawada, T. et al. (2009). Whole body bioimpedance monitoring for outpatient chronic heart failure follow up. *Circulation Journal, 73,* 1074–1079.

Wagner, D.R. & Heyward, V.H. (1999). Techniques of body composition assessment: a review of laboratory and field methods. *Research Quarterly for Exercise and Sport, 70,* 135–149.

4

PHYSIQUE: PHENOTYPE, SOMATOTYPE AND 3D SCANNING

J.E. Lindsay Carter and Arthur D. Stewart

This chapter will cover:

4.1 Introduction to the human phenotype
4.2 Somatotype definitions and components
4.3 The anthropometric and photoscopic somatotype methods
4.4 The emergence of 3D photonic scanning
4.5 The human phenotype today

4.1 Introduction to the human phenotype

Visual observations of the human body form are instinctively based on general characteristics. The whole human body is a *phenotype*, which constitutes the visible properties of an organism arising from the interaction of the genotype and the environment. The characteristics evaluated in the human organism depend upon what we are looking for and the methods used in the observations. Much of modern medicine and physiology is concerned only with quantifying fatness, ignoring other parameters which determine overall morphology. This chapter considers these often overlooked variables, and the contribution they can make to our understanding of health and performance.

Scientific measurement of human physique and body types has a long history dating back to the father of modern medicine, Hippocrates (*c*.460–370 BC), who formally classified bodies into two fundamental body types in the fifth century BC as 'appoplecticus' and 'phthiscus'. In the 1820s, Léon Rostan (1790–1866), a reknowned medical scholar, identified 'digestif', 'musculaire' and cérébral'. In the 1920s, Ernst Kretschmer (1888–1964) a psychiatrist interested in the link between personality and morphology, identified 'pyknic' (fat) 'athletic' (muscular) and 'asthenic' (thin) types. Later, other scientists developed categorical classifications of physique ranging from two to five 'types' (Tucker & Lessa, 1940). Much as we can applaud the effort of their approaches to recognise the variability introduced by muscularity and frame size in addition to adiposity, these discrete categories were very general and limited because not everyone could be placed accurately within them. Further, the lack of a universal typology limited its acceptance within the scientific and medical communities.

Two major methods of assessing the whole body phenotype are in current use: *somatotyping* and *whole body 3D photonic scanning*. The current methods of somatotyping have been in use for over 40 years, but methods for 3D scanning are more recent and have undergone great progress since the turn of the millennium. The somatotype may be obtained by simple anthropometry, ratings of a three-view photograph, or a combination of the two. Anthropometry, as defined in Chapter 3, is a suitable classroom, field or laboratory method for rating the somatotype. Photonic scanning requires expensive equipment and expertise but has added new perspectives on how we measure and evaluate physiques. Scanning in three dimensions can not only obtain the contour of the body surface, but cross-sectional areas and volumes in addition, to derive a full topography of the body shape. In a similar way to photography being the developing technology of the early twentieth century, 3D scanning represents the equivalent of the twenty-first.

We live in an expanding universe of possible physique types and both methods have their place. The somatotype offers the best objective quantification of a total physique and is the yardstick for describing populations and in aesthetic or body image applications. These now can be extended by new scanning technologies. Both methods summarise the physique in a comprehensive whole body manner which overcomes major weakness in studies which use simplistic variables such as body mass index (BMI), etc. Assessment of the phenotype by either method allows for monitoring stability or change under the influences of growth and ageing, exercise, training and performance, diet and nutrition, and behaviour. Current methods of somatotyping and 3D scanning are reviewed in the following sections.

Somatotype

Somatotyping is a method for describing the human physique in terms of a number of traits that relate to body shape and composition. The result is the holistic or phenotypical somatotype. The somatotype gives an overall summary of the physique as a unified whole. Its utility is in the combination of three aspects of physique into a somatotype rating. It combines the appraisal of adiposity, musculo-skeletal robustness and linearity into the three-numbered rating and conjures up a visual image of the three aspects of the physique.

Sheldon, Stephens & Tucker (1940) introduced a classic approach that led to today's commonly used method. In Sheldon's method an attempt was made to describe the genotypical morphological traits of a person in terms of three components, each on a seven-point scale. This genotypic approach, the rigidity of the closed seven-point ratings and a lack of objectivity of the ratings, made the method unattractive to most researchers, especially in the fields of body composition and kinanthropometry.

Essentially, Sheldon claimed that the adult somatotype in the early twenties was "fixed" for life and that changes in physique did not alter the rating for males younger or older. He did no longitudinal studies to support this view, but developed age-group sliding scales to 'prove' his claim. In response to criticism he developed a new method, the *Trunk Index*, which involved planimetry of the upper and lower trunk as well as new tables for somatotypes and stature. This 'index' method only confused matters and was not accepted by most investigators who were more concerned with the phenotype and recording change in physique and body composition from infancy to old age for both males and females. Several authors made modifications to the Sheldon method while attempting to objectively rate various samples. Hooton (1951), Dupertuis & Emanuel (1956) and Damon (1955) studied military personnel; Bullen & Hardy (1946) derived a checklist for rating female somatotypes; and Parnell (1954, 1958) developed the M.4 Deviation Chart which made ratings more objective for children and adults of both genders. These and other authors showed that there were differences between methods and that it was important to state the somatotype method used in studies. Clearly, there was a need for a more universal method of somatotyping. Comparisons between methods are summarised in Carter & Heath (1990, pp. 70–72).

In the 1960s a new and more 'universal phenotype' method by Heath (1963) and Heath & Carter (1967) emerged. It was largely influenced by ideas from Parnell (1954, 1958) and Heath's rejection of the genotypic approach which she learned when working with Sheldon in the 1950s. Heath & Carter adopted this phenotypic approach, with open rating scales for three components and ratings that can be estimated from objective anthropometric measurements and photoscopic rating criteria. The Heath-Carter somatotype method is currently the most universally applied, and is described below. Extensive descriptions of the method, its development and applications, can be found in Carter & Ackland (2009), Carter & Heath (1990), and Duquet & Carter (2009).

4.2 Somatotype definitions and components

The somatotype is a quantified expression or description of the present morphological conformation of a person. It always consists of a three-numeral rating, for example, 3½-5-1. The three numerals are always recorded in the same order, endomorphy, mesomorphy and ectomorphy (defined below), each describing the value of a particular component of physique. The somatotype tells the observer what kind of physique an individual has and how it looks (Duquet & Carter, 2009). Ratings on each component of ½ to 2½ are considered low, 3 to 5 are moderate, 5½ to 7 are high, and 7½ and above are very high. The component scales have an observed range from ½ to 16+ for endomorphy, ½ to 12+ for mesomorphy, and ½ to 9+ for ectomorphy. That is, the high end of the scales are open-ended and could go beyond the upper ratings if warranted by the data. The rating is phenotypical, based on the concept of geometrical size-dissociation and applicable to both genders from childhood to old age. The rating is independent of stature so can be used across the age span (Carter & Heath, 1990).

Components

A component is an empirically defined descriptor of a particular aspect or trait of the human body build. It is expressed as a numeral on a continuous scale, which theoretically starts at zero and has no upper limit. The ratings are rounded to the half-unit. In practice, no ratings lower than ½ are given (as a particular body build trait can never be absolutely absent), and a rating of more than 7 is extremely high.

Endomorphy

The first component, called endomorphy, describes the relative degree of adiposity of the body, regardless of where or how it is distributed. It also describes corresponding physical aspects, such as roundness of the body, softness of the contours, relative volume of the abdominal trunk and distally tapering of the limbs.

Mesomorphy

The second component, called mesomorphy, describes the relative musculo-skeletal development of the body. It also describes corresponding physical aspects, such as the apparent robustness of the body in terms of muscle or bone, the relative volume of the thoracic trunk and the possibility of hidden muscle bulk.

The definitions of endomorphy and mesomorphy reflect the anatomical model of body composition.

Ectomorphy

The third component, called ectomorphy, describes the relative slenderness of the body. It also describes corresponding physical aspects, such as the relative linearity of the body or fragility of the limbs, in absence of any bulk, be it muscle, adipose or other tissues.

The following description of the Heath-Carter somatotype method is adapted from Carter & Ackland (2009).

There are three methods for obtaining the somatotype.

- The *anthropometric* method, in which body measurements are used to estimate the criterion somatotype.
- The *photoscopic* method, in which ratings by criterion raters are made from a standardised photograph of front, side and back views, taken in minimal clothing, as illustrated in Figure 4.1.
- The *anthropometric plus photoscopic* method, which combines anthropometry and ratings from a photograph – which is considered to be the criterion method.

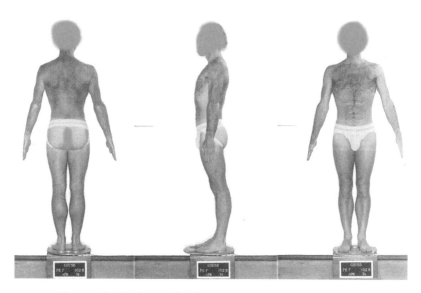

FIGURE 4.1 The standardised pose for the somatotype photograph. The subject is a 42-year-old male whose photoscopic somatotype rating is: 2-5-3.

4.3 The anthropometric and photoscopic somatotype methods

Because most researchers lack the opportunity to become a criterion somatotype rater using photographs, the anthropometric method has emerged as the most useful for a wide variety of applications.

The anthropometric somatotype rating form

Ten anthropometric dimensions are needed to calculate the anthropometric somatotype: stretch stature, body mass, four skinfolds (triceps, subscapular, supraspinale, medial calf), two bone breadths (biepicondylar humerus and femur), and two limb girths (arm flexed and tensed, calf). These measurements are taken according to the International Society for the Advancement of Kinanthropometry standard (Stewart, Marfell-Jones, Olds & de Ridder, 2011) or Carter & Ackland (2009) and entered into the rating form to calculate the somatotype, following the descriptions in Carter & Ackland (2009), Carter & Heath (1990) or Duquet & Carter (2009). Examples of completed rating forms are contained in these latter three references.

The anthropometric somatotype rating form is useful for teaching students as well as individual assessment of clients. It helps users to understand the concepts and which measures contribute to the somatotype and is also useful to check for errors in measurement. Note that in the mesomorphy section, when obtained values are outside the columns at the low or high end, additional columns must be extrapolated beyond the values in the rating form.

The anthropometric somatotype equations

The second method of obtaining the anthropometric somatotype components is by means of equations into which the ten measurements are entered. Equations can be used for individual or group calculations and are in more common use than the rating form. For individual interpretation, the decimal components are usually rounded to the nearest half-unit.

$$Endomorphy = -0.7182 + 0.1451 \, (X) - 0.00068 \, (X^2) + 0.0000014 \, (X^3)$$

where $X =$ (sum of triceps, subscapular and supraspinale skinfolds) multiplied by (170.18 / stature in cm). This 'height-corrected endomorphy' and is the preferred method for calculating endomorphy.

$$Mesomorphy = 0.858 \times humerus \; breadth + 0.601 \times femur \; breadth + \\ 0.188 \times corrected \; arm \; girth + 0.161 \times corrected \; calf \; girth - height \; 0.131 + 4.5.$$

[N.B. corrected arm girth = arm girth flexed and tensed minus triceps skinfold in cm; corrected calf girth = calf girth minus calf skinfold in cm.]

Three different equations are used to calculate *ectomorphy* according to the height-weight ratio*:

If HWR is greater than or equal to 40.75, then *ectomorphy* = 0.732 HWR - 28.58

If HWR is less than 40.75 but greater than 38.25, then *ectomorphy* = 0.463 HWR - 17.63

If HWR is equal to or less than 38.25, then *ectomorphy* = 0.1

*The height-weight ratio (HWR), or stature divided by the cube root of mass (i.e. $stature/mass^{1/3}$), as used in somatotyping.

The preceding equations use metric units. The equation for endomorphy is a third degree polynomial. The equations for mesomorphy and ectomorphy are linear. If the equation calculation for any component is zero or negative, a value of 0.1 is assigned as the component rating, because by definition ratings cannot be zero or negative.

Photoscopic somatotype

The photoscopic somatotype should only be rated objectively by persons who have trained to attain the necessary skill, and whose rating validity and reliability is established against those of an experienced rater. It is, however, generally accepted that the anthropometric evaluation gives a fairly good estimate (~90 per cent agreement) of the photoscopic procedure. Important deviations are only found in subjects with high amounts of, or with dysplasia in, adipose or muscle tissue. Many researchers, who do not use photographs or visual inspection, or who lack experience in rating photoscopically, report the anthropometric somatotype only. The criterion somatotype method is the combination of both methods, and is rarely used. As a consequence, when reporting a somatotype, researchers should always state the method employed. In order to help with interpretation of the numerical somatotype values, the characteristics associated with each component and values in the rating scales are shown in Figure 4.2.

The Heath-Carter photoscopic somatotype

PHOTOSCOPIC SOMATOTYPE RATING FORM

1. ENDOMORPHY RATING SCALE AND CHARACTERISTICS (Relative adiposity)

1 1½ 2 2½	3 3½ 4 4½ 5	5½ 6 6½ 7	7½ 8 8½ 9......
Low relative adiposity; little subcutaneous fat; muscle and bone outlines visible.	Moderate relative adiposity; subcutaneous fat covers muscle and bone outlines; softer appearance.	High relative adiposity; thick subcutaneous fat; roundness of trunk and limbs; increased storage of fat in abdomen.	Extremely high relative adiposity; very thick subcutaneous fat and high amounts of abdominal trunk fat; proximal concentration of fat in limbs.

2. MESOMORPHY RATING SCALE AND CHARACTERISTICS (Musculo-skeletal robustness relative to height)

1 1½ 2 2½	3 3½ 4 4½ 5	5½ 6 6½ 7	7½ 8 8½ 9......
Low relative musculo-skeletal development; narrow skeletal diameters; narrow muscle diameters; small joints in limbs.	Moderate relative musculo-skeletal development; increased muscle bulk and thicker bones and joints.	High relative musculo-skeletal development; wide skeletal diameters; bulky muscles; large joints.	Extremely high relative musculo-skeletal development; very bulky muscles; very wide skeleton and joints.

3. ECTOMORPHY RATING SCALE AND CHARACTERISTICS (Relative linearity)

1 1½ 2 2½	3 3½ 4 4½ 5	5½ 6 6½ 7	7½ 8 8½ 9......
Low relative linearity; great bulk per unit of height; round like a ball; relatively bulky limbs.	Moderate relative linearity; less bulk per unit of height; more stretched-out.	High relative linearity; little bulk per unit of height.	Extremely high relative linearity; very stretched-out; narrow like a pencil; minimal bulk per unit of height

PHOTOSCOPIC RATING INFORMATION

I.D. ....Name..Age..........   Male ....Female.......Date...................

Height..............Weight..................HWR................... First estimate.................. Final rating...................

NOTES:..

FIGURE 4.2 Photoscopic somatotype rating form. This form is used along with the photoscopic criteria and reference photographs to help establish the rating for each component. The written descriptions can be used to explain the anthropometric and/or photoscopic somatotype rating.

Plotting the somatotype: the somatochart

Traditionally, the three–number somatotype rating is plotted on a two-dimensional somatochart using XY coordinates derived from the rating (see Figure 4.3). The coordinates are calculated as follows:

$$X = ectomorphy - endomorphy$$
$$Y = 2 \times mesomorphy - (endomorphy + ectomorphy)$$

The male participant in Figure 4.1, together with the female participant depicted in the 3D scanner (in Figure 4.5) are illustrated as points on the somatochart called somatoplots, in Figure 4.3. If the somatoplot for any participant is far from that expected when compared to a suitable reference group, it is important to check the data and calculations. Somatocharts with or without the printed somatotype numbers can be also be used and are available from Goulding (2010).

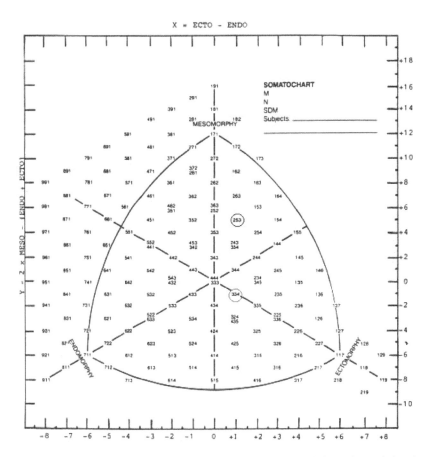

FIGURE 4.3 Somatoplot of the male participant in Figure 4.1 (dark circle) and also the female participant in 3D scanning (Figure 4.5).

Somatotype categories

A somatotype category is the more qualitative verbal description of the individual somatotype, in terms of the dominant component or components. For example, a subject with a high rating on mesomorphy and an equally low rating on endomorphy and ectomorphy, will be called a Mesomorph, or more precisely a balanced Mesomorph. A subject with dominant endomorphy and mesomorphy greater than ectomorphy will be called a mesomorphic Endomorph. For help with language translations it is recommended that the three components as nouns, Endomorph, Mesomorphy and Ectomorph, be written with the first letter as a capital. The lesser components are adjectives and are written with a lower case first letter. If two components are equal, both first letters are capitalised.

The definitions of 13 categories are based on the areas of the 2D somatochart (adapted from Carter & Heath, 1990).

- *Central*: no component differs by more than one unit from the other two.
- *balanced Endomorph*: endomorphy is dominant and mesomorphy and ectomorphy are equal (or do not differ by more than one-half unit).
- *mesomorphic Endomorph*: endomorphy is dominant and mesomorphy is greater than ectomorphy.
- *Mesomorph-Endomorph*: endomorphy and mesomorphy are equal (or do not differ by more than one-half unit), and ectomorphy is smaller.
- *endomorphic Mesomorph*: mesomorphy is dominant and endomorphy is greater than ectomorphy.
- *balanced Mesomorph*: mesomorphy is dominant and endomorphy and ectomorphy are equal (or do not differ by more than one-half unit).
- *ectomorphic Mesomorph*: mesomorphy is dominant and ectomorphy is greater than endomorphy.
- *Mesomorph-Ectomorph*: mesomorphy and ectomorphy are equal (or do not differ by more than one-half unit), and endomorphy is smaller.
- *mesomorphic Ectomorph*: ectomorphy is dominant and mesomorphy is greater than endomorphy.
- *balanced Ectomorph*: ectomorphy is dominant and endomorphy and mesomorphy are equal (or do not differ by more than one-half unit).
- *endomorphic Ectomorph*: ectomorphy is dominant and endomorphy is greater than mesomorphy.
- *Endomorph-Ectomorph*: endomorphy and ectomorphy are equal (or do not differ by more than one-half unit), and mesomorphy is lower.
- *ectomorphic Endomorph*: endomorphy is dominant and ectomorphy is greater than mesomorphy.

The 13 categories can be simplified into four larger categories:

- *Central*: no component differs by more than one unit from the other two.

- *Endomorph*: endomorphy is dominant, mesomorphy and ectomorphy are more than one-half unit lower.
- *Mesomorph*: mesomorphy is dominant, endomorphy and ectomorphy are more than one-half unit lower.
- *Ectomorph*: ectomorphy is dominant, endomorphy and mesomorphy are more than one-half unit lower.

The three-dimensional somatotype

Because the somatotype is a three-number expression, meaningful analyses can be conducted only with special techniques. The three component scales are on three perpendicular axes, x, y and z (akin to the edges of a box). Somatotype data can be analysed by both traditional and non-traditional descriptive and comparative statistical methods Although descriptive statistics are used for each of the components, comparative statistics should be made in the first instance using the whole (or 'global') somatotype rating. This is normally followed by analysis of separate components. These analyses are described in Duquet & Carter (2009). Here are some further definitions which are useful in this respect:

A *somatopoint* (S) is a point in three-dimensional space determined from the somatotype which is represented by a triad of x, y and z coordinates for the three components. The scales on the coordinate axes are component units with the hypothetical somatotype 0-0-0 at the origin of the three axes.

The *somatotype attitudinal distance* (SAD) is the distance in three dimensions between any two somatopoints, calculated in component units.

The *somatotype attitudinal mean* (SAM) is the average of the SADs of each somatopoint from the mean somatopoint (S) of a sample.

The SAD represents the 'true' distance between two somatopoints (A and B). The SAD is calculated as follows:

$$SAD\ (A;B) = \sqrt{[(end(A) - end(B))^2 + (mes(A) - mes(B))^2 + (ect(A) - ect(B))^2]}$$

$$SAM = \Sigma\ SADi\ /\ N_x$$

where: SAD = Somatotype Attitudinal Distance; SAM = Somatotype Attitudinal Mean; end = endomorphy rating; mes = mesomorphy rating; ect = ectomorphy rating; A = an individual or a group; B = an individual or a group; N_x = number of subjects in group X.

Further information about the somatotype and programs for statistics and plotting, is available from Golding (2010).

There are a range of applications of the somatotype, including psychiatry and psychological research, body image assessment, growth and development, sports talent identification, and to describe the phenotype associated with several clinical pathologies. Since the 1960 Rome Olympics, which included a large systematic measurement survey of Olympic athletes (Tanner, 1964), the recognition of the different physique types in different athletic disciplines have been widely appreciated. This can help identify the distinctiveness of physiques associated with different sporting disciplines, and whether a competitive gradient exists in physique variation. Readers are referred to Carter & Heath (1990) for a comprehensive treatment of different studies of somatotype of individual sports, growth and ageing.

Somatotype studies continue in a variety of topics and across many countries. In addition to the study of female basketball players (Carter, Ackland, Kerr & Stapff, 2005), there are many studies on a variety of sports, such as on soccer and volleyball (Bandyopadhyay, 2007), rugby (Holway & Garavaglia, 2009), and power lifters (Keogh, Hume, Pearson & Mellow, 2007). Growth studies have been carried out in India (Gaur, Maurya & Kang, 2008), South Africa (Makgae, Monyeki, Brits, Kemper & Mashita, 2007), and Bulgaria (Mladenovam Nikolova, Andreenko & Boyadjiev2010). Also, there are interesting population studies with different approaches as shown by Ghosh & Malik (2010) on Santhals in India, (Rebato, Jelenkovic & Salces, 2007) and by Saranga et al. (2008) who studied hereditability in Biscay and Mozambique populations respectively.

Somatotype and 3D scanning

An early attempt to augment somatotyping, had it been pursued, might been the forerunner of current 3D scanning. Preston & Singh (1972) proposed a modification of somatotype methods by introducing 'redintegrated somatotyping'. This involved integrating photographic diameters of limbs and torso with height, and using photoelectronic computation and analysis, to produce graphical representations which were exact (though possibly meaningless) quantifications, more indicative of issues of body surface measurement than to somatotyping. The somatotype photograph and 3D scanning are similar in that they both show the present morphology of the subject as seen from the 'outside'. They show how the physique looks. If skinfolds, girths and breadths are taken for the anthropometric somatotype, some underlying tissues can be differentiated. In 3D scans areas and volumes can be derived, but not tissue composition. It is often interesting to observe dysplasia, which is bad shape or form, in physiques. In somatotyping it refers to disharmony or uneven distribution of a component or components in different anatomical regions of the body. Dysplasia is often seen as greater endomorphy or mesomorphy in the upper versus lower half of the body (or vice versa). Comparing upper and lower body parts in terms of cross-sections and volumes from 3D scans can also provide estimates of dysplasia. The development of 3D scanning as a technique can provide more quantitative estimates of dysplasia than limited anthropometry or somatotype photographs.

4.4 The emergence of 3D photonic scanning

Three-dimensional photonic scanning enables profiling of the body in unprecedented ways. Its development over the past 25 years for the clothing and automotive industries has included approaches using (A) structured light, (B) class 1 (eye-safe) lasers or (C) millimetre wave technologies. These have made contributions to epidemiological research and, more recently, sports and exercise science.

Structured light can be projected onto the body to produce patterns which are distorted by the body surface contour and captured by cameras (e.g. InSpeck, Wicks and Wilson, TC²). Linear array millimetre radio wave technology has the capability of scanning through clothing and uses a moveable wand that rotates around the body (e.g. Intellifit). Class 1 (eye-safe) lasers enable triangulation of data points to capture shape (e.g. Cyberware, Hamamatsu, Human Solutions). An example of a laser scanner is illustrated in Figure 4.4. All approaches measure the body non-invasively, with rapid throughput producing dimensions of interest for

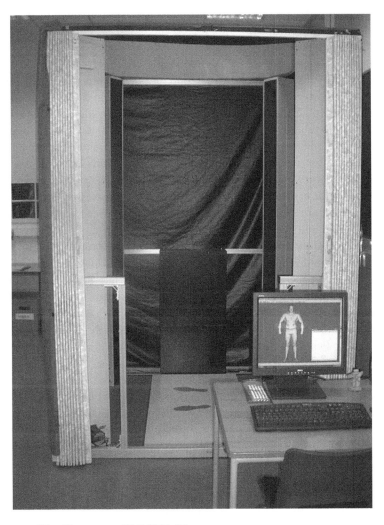

FIGURE 4.4 The Hamamatsu BLS 9036–02 scanner.

a range of applications. Once the primary measurement data are obtained, subsequent analysis can be performed using system software, which can produce output in a range of file formats. Images are captured initially as point cloud data, where approaching one million points can represent the human body in xyz space. Software processing tools enable the image to undergo primary landmarking, where easily located landmarks such as the vertex, C7, axilla and crotch are input, from which system software performs a rendering of a 3D textured mesh with evenly spaced points, which is segmented into distinct regions. Secondary landmarking derives landmarks from the primary points using sophisticated computer techniques such as salient point detection or curve estimation, but alternatively these can be manually placed prior to scanning or digitally placed during analysis. Capturing the body in a standard pose, very similar to the somatotype pose (but with feet farther apart) may involve some shadowing whereby the skin surface is obscured and missing data result. Also, reflective colours, or jewellery cause data loss and approaches to standardise clothing are necessary. Hole-filling software is available to complete a fully rendered shape for export, although different scan software systems appear reasonably resilient at rendering meshes with some missing data. The prospect of visualisation of the body in a novel way and rapid prototyping – the construction of a 3D model using synthetic materials, based on the 3D data file – opens up a range of possibilities by which the phenotype of the individual can be used. While the driver for much of the technological advancement has been the animations industry, the multidisciplinary nature of 3D data and the use to which they may be put has enabled cross-talk between disciplines in an unprecedented way, the result of which has been an exciting range of works within the realms of health, sport and beyond.

One principal attraction for using 3D scanning in place of surface anthropometry is that it can capture body shape, without physically touching the participant, in much less time. The participant, wearing light-coloured, form-fitting clothing, stands inside the scanning chamber and assumes a standard pose for the 10–15 seconds required for the scan. After the scan is analysed, the digital shape file affords the opportunity to quantify body dimensions retrospectively. These features lend the scanning technology an advantage for survey work where a rapid throughput of individuals is required.

'While 3D whole body scanning has a number of limitations relative to traditional surface anthropometry – expense, technical expertise required, inability to take skinfolds and compressed bone breadths – it offers an opportunity to collect much greater volumes of data without the subject being present during the measurement. It also expands the types of measurements that can be made into two and three dimensions. It captures anthropometric data in a form which can be fed into and used by new and powerful software applications in areas such as ergonomics and apparel design'.

(Olds & Honey 2006, p. 12)

While 3D scanning does have advantages over anthropometry – notably measurement and analysis times as well as cross-sectional areas and segmental volumes, the differences between the approaches are important to appreciate. These are summarised in Table 4.1.

TABLE 4.1 Comparison of surface anthropometry and 3D scanning

	Surface anthropometry	3D scanning
Skeletal lengths and breadths	✓	✓ (approximated, because no compression of overlying tissues)
Direct surface distances	✓	✓
Assessment of subcutaneous adipose tissue	✓	✗
Girths	✓	✓
Cross sectional areas	✗	✓
Segmental volumes	✗	✓
Measurement time	45 minutes for a full profile	10–15 seconds
Analysis time	10 minutes	1–5 minutes
Key advantages	Standardised procedures True skeletal dimensions Global acceptance	Speed of data acquisition link to other analytical tools Re-analysis capability
Disadvantages	Training essential for reliable measurements Time consuming	Cost, availability, No globally accepted procedures Clothing colour, hirsutism can influence output

Three-dimensional photonic scanning data have been used to illustrate how males and females differ fundamentally in BMI-shape relationships (Wells, Treleaven & Cole, 2007). This study resulted from the Size UK clothing survey whereby a consortium of retailers in collaboration with University College London, surveyed adults 9,617 adults aged between 16 and 91 years, across eight cities. Their objective was to update the design templates for clothing with the actual shapes of a representative sample of UK adults, but the data set is so comprehensive, it can be interpreted in many ways from a health perspective. This is important, because scanning can capture girths which can be used directly or as ratios to assign health risk. These are discussed in more detail in Chapter 7, but it has long been recognised that an enlarged waist girth is linked with cardiovascular disease (Ducimetiere,

Richard & Cambian, 1986) and type 2 diabetes (Björntorp, 1988), while enlarged thigh fat is considered protective of health (Kahn, Austin, Williamson & Arensberg, 1996), as it offers an alternative storage location which appears to avoid the same risk. An interesting question here relates to whether or not the waist should be expected to increase as a direct proportion to stature, following the law of geometric similarity. Considering the size of the skeleton and internal organs being larger with increased stature, this might seem a logical assumption. However, the data in the study of Wells and colleagues show the waist in males to have a negative correlation with height, a finding that the authors attributed to genetics or a link between early growth and a predisposition to obesity. This view is supported by observations of critical periods in growth relating to the 'adiposity rebound' (Cameron & Demerath, 2002). This associates an early nadir of BMI and fat in mid childhood to increased adiposity in adolescence and early adulthood, which, along with related issues, will be discussed in greater detail in Chapter 8. An alternative explanation offered by Nevill, Stewart & Olds (2010) was that the smaller skeleton of shorter men has less ability to accommodate increasing fatness without expanding the waist. While this might be a statement of the obvious, it has cast further doubt on the utility of BMI to describe shape, especially in a health context, where more than a little controversially, it endures as the metric to describe obesity and public health. Further detail on the use and limitations of BMI is covered in Chapter 7. The retailers who sponsored the survey were also interested in the age variability in shape for any given size, and the study was able to quantify this using data which were subsequently used to produce age-specific dressmakers' dummies for the appropriate shape at a given clothing size.

The effect of age on physique was strong in women, but not men (Wells, Cole & Treleaven, 2008a). Increasing age was associated with increased bust and waist girths, but decreased thigh girth, and while younger obese women maintained an hourglass figure, older obese women had shapes more similar to men. Conversely, obese men had similar shapes across different age categories. The authors postulated that the age-delay in the association between obesity and high waist girth in women may partly explain the difference in life expectancy between men and women. However, there are inevitable limitations of such a cross-sectional design, so interpretation is necessarily prudent. A further development of the analysis of clothing survey data for health application was the comparison of the UK data with a multi-ethnic sample from the USA (Wells, Cole, Bruner & Treleaven, 2008b). This was a study with important implications, because the rates of obesity are higher amongst Hispanic and African Americans than whites. They identified gradients relating morphology to socio-economic and educational status, showing that in white and Hispanic Americans, increasing status was directly associated with height. In white and African Americans, increased status was inversely proportional to waist. Comparing the white Britons and Americans, adjusted for age and height, Americans had greater girths, BMI and weight than their UK counterparts. Comparison of girths revealed highly significant inter-ethnic differences at all girths. While it has been established that Asians are known to have increased fatness and disease risk at a given level of BMI compared with Europeans, the study showed the populations differences in BMI did not correspond to shape differences. Specifically, African American men were heavier than whites, but had smaller waist and larger thigh girths. Hispanic men and women had larger waists and smaller thighs, yet lower BMI than whites. The pattern of shape variability closely tracks the pattern of metabolic syndrome observed in different ethnic groups. Taken together, the 3D scan data can make a considerable contribution to such epidemiological research, as a direct consequence of the utility and capability for large surveys which have the power to detect morphological differences which are important determinants of health.

Comparison of a 1950s anthropometric clothing survey and the recent size survey show UK women to have gained an average 4 cm in stature, 4 cm in hip girth and 14 cm in waist measurements. This clearly implies a substantial shape change, although this finding assumes equivalence between anthropometric and 3D methods. Locating the anatomical waist is straightforward in an 'hourglass' figure, but a convex profile it is more problematic and may require landmarking. Different protocols use slightly different approaches to this which can limit the validity of comparing data from different sources. This was noted using anthropometric protocols which produced results which differed by up to 5.4 per cent and 1.7 per cent in women and men respectively (Wang et al., 2003). Using the digital capability of the 3D scanning technique, the variability within the waist region (inferior of the tenth rib and superior to the iliac crest) was quantified as 11.4 per cent and 4.9 per cent in women and men respectively (Stewart, Nevill, Stephen & Young, 2010). This is a potentially important difference, because using conventional anthropometry, serial measures will not necessarily capture the same posture or position in the ventilatory cycle, whereas the retrospective measurement of the 3D scan can use the same raw data file to make such a comparison.

As mentioned in Chapter 2, the 3D scanning method has also been validated for assessing body volume and percentage fat prediction (Wang et al., 2006). In this study, 44 females and 48 males representing a wide range of age and size were assessed both by 3D photonic scanning and anthropometry. Of these, 63 were assessed using densitometry, with residual lung volume measured. The 3D measures were slightly but significantly greater than those using manual anthropometry or densitometry-derived volume. The authors note that the 3D girth measures are constrained to the horizontal plane, and the difficulty which some volunteers might experience attempting to exhale maximally and stand motionless for the ten seconds duration of the scan. Despite the slight difference in measures between densitometry and 3D scanning, when converted into percentage fat the differences were not significant. The authors did conclude that accurate volume measures were possible using 3D scanning if appropriate clothing was worn and the protocol was adhered to. Considering the large individual variability in some of their participants, which in some cases predicts percentage body fat higher by 3D scanning by over 20 per cent, it is less reliable than the more established laboratory techniques discussed in Chapter 2.

Because male and female data are not presented separately, the effect of hirsutism, which might explain the enlarged girths and volumes of some individuals measured by 3D scanning, cannot be quantified. Because the 3D scanning approach involves the triangulation of points at the outermost tip of the measured surface, individuals with significant body hair are likely to find enlarged values. While Chapter 2 underlines the limitations of densitometry being considered a reference technique for determining percentage fat, it is considered the method of choice for determining body volume. In a different study, 3D laser scans were compared with manual anthropometry and DXA scanning for assessment of fatness in US Army personnel (Garlie, Obusek, Corner & Zambraski, 2010). Their study involved 37 male participants whose BMI ranged between 20 and 32.5 kg.m^{-2}, who were assessed on a Cyberware WB4 scanner (Cyberware, Inc. Monterey, CA, USA) and a Lunar Prodigy DXA scanner (GE Medical Systems, USA). Percentage fat was calculated using the Army's prediction based on a logarithmic computation of abdominal and neck girths and stature calculated from manual and 3D measurements. This study also included correcting errors in automated landmarking introduced by the software in a small number of cases, although the instructions for breathing for the 3D scanning were not specified. The lack of difference between DXA, 3D and anthropometry-derived fat estimates seems encouraging, and the use of the girths rather than volume to produce estimates of fatness might explain the findings and pave the way for further research on fat estimates based on a greater number of girths. However, this study also illustrates that 3D and DXA scanning share the commonality of 'undisclosed algorithms' for locating measurements in 3D, and assuming fat distribution in DXA, both of which yield unquantified error which future research must address.

The requirement for participants to wear form-fitting clothing – which can be a severe limitation in obesity or body image research – is no impediment for research with athletes, many of whom are required to wear such clothing in training and competition. To date, no study assessing body fatness in athletes via 3D scanning has been undertaken, because of the limited availability of scanning facilities. However, recent access to this technology by elite athletes has enabled quantification of body segments amongst rowers, which has produced data (such as segmental volumes) which are clearly significant, but which could not have been assessed using conventional anthropometry. This study quantified the variation for these dimensions in light and heavyweight rowers and how these differ from the general population in terms of effect size and variability (Schranz, Tomkinson, Olds & Daniell, 2010). Unsurprisingly, heavyweight rowers were much larger than the general population, and lightweight rowers similar or smaller, but rowers had dimensions which were less variable. This study was the first of its kind and usefully quantifies the physique specialisation required for lightweight and heavyweight quantified for both males and females. Although it did not attempt to quantify minimum weight or fatness, but is a potentially useful adjunct to existing measures, which may be pertinent in weight-restricted sports. Furthermore, the rapid profiling enables greater numbers of athletes to be surveyed within the limitations of time and cost, and its combination with other measurement modalities will undoubtedly represent a major advance in future body composition research.

4.5 The human phenotype today

It might at first seem that the phenotype just 'happens' as a consequence of functional adaptation. However, the reality is far from the truth. A range of behaviours result from the phenotype, which are manifest in social interaction. At puberty, we see the clear sexual dimorphism which prevails throughout life, though it diminishes somewhat in later years. As well as fulfilling the different functions of males and females, the phenotype has a unique role in sexual attractiveness and partner selection. Biologically, female animals compete with one another to attract males by effectively advertising their reproductive potential. In humans this is commonly associated with a youthful appearance, where fat patterning depicts and emphasises certain aspects of shape such as breast profile and waist curvature. Male animal attractiveness is seen, in biological terms as conveying dominance, and the capability of intimidating other males. While behavioural and cultural parameters have equally powerful effects in humans, the morphological basis for recognising attractiveness still prevails.

An interesting observation is that there is also a culturally specific effect which appears to be at work here. In some cultures, obesity and overweight is seen as a sign of wealth. In the UK, a trend analysis was conducted on the data of over 500 *Playboy* centrefold models, whose data on height, weight, bust, waist and hip girth were reported between 1953 and 2001 (Voracek & Fisher, 2002). This followed a similar line of enquiry as previous research on shop mannequins, which questioned whether there was a fashion for a certain physique profile. Their data showed clearly that there were highly significant temporal trends for BMI to decline, waist to hip ratio and *androgyny index* [waist / (hip × bust)$^{0.5}$] to increase suggesting that such models are becoming less hourglass shaped and more ectomorphic over time. As these data coincide with the comparative data from the previous clothing survey and the more recent Size UK survey, the reference female population has also exhibited a trend in shape. However, this trend, rather than tracking such linearity, does the reverse. As such, the gap between the typical shape and the perceived ideal shape appears to be widening. This is a worrying trend, because overweight and obesity are associated with a diminished body image and greater dissatisfaction.

Males and females clearly express different levels of dissatisfaction in different anatomical regions with males generally seeking larger, and females seeking smaller size in most body regions (Stewart, Giles, Johnstone & Benson, 2008). This mismatch of desired and actual physique has contributed to the development of eating disorders, and is not helped by the media's role in portraying the idealised super-slim female or bodybuilder male as aspirational, though for most individuals, unattainable. Furthermore, the observation that eating disordered patients tend to perceive their true shape less accurately than those of a healthy weight has also been recognised in obese individuals (Johnstone et al., 2008). In this connection, somatotype offers a useful metric for quantifying physique preference, because it conveys objectively the actual physique against which other parameters can be measured (Stewart, Benson, Michanikou, Tsiota & Narli, 2003). However, due to fat accumulation occurring in sex and age specific patterns, there is scope for 3D views of the body (as opposed to the traditional three-pose photograph) providing additional information in this regard, an example of which is illustrated in Figure 4.5. Pilot work using 3D scanning in anorexic and bulimic patients has identified different area:volume relationships from controls, and has established the viability of this approach in future clinical trials (Stewart et al., 2012).

As things currently stand, most of the developmental work using 3D scanning has been carried out in the computer graphics and animations industries. A good example of this is a landmark paper by Allen, Curless & Popović (2003). This models a series of 3D scans to synthesize digital characters which can be transferred and 'skeletonised' for animation. This approach is being used increasingly in the film industry for digital effect creation which has the dual benefit of enhanced capability and reduced cost resulting from fewer 'extras' being required for crowd scenes etc. This capability combines the finer points of 3D shape, complex algorithms for movement and very large computing power. This same combination has the potential to inform other areas of research too. For instance, consider the challenge the female body is faced with in late pregnancy, in maintaining posture, balance and locomotion while a systematic shape and mass change take place. Additional fat accumulation typically follows a gluteo-femoral distribution, and it has been previously suggested that this counterbalances the anterior development of the abdomen to overcome the threat to stability (Pawlowski, 2001). Whereas a typical android distribution would further destabilise the pregnant female, a gynoid distribution preserves equilibrium and distributes forces along the spinal column. Without such a counterbalance effect, basic locomotion and foraging would have

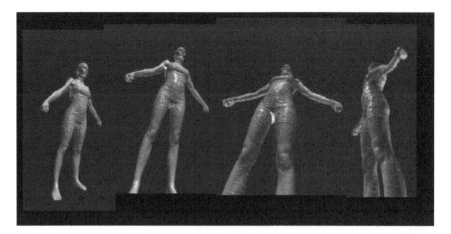

FIGURE 4.5 Example of a control participant's 3D scan as viewed from a visualisation software application, developed for body image applications.

created additional risks for survival in our evolutionary past. While this theory may be logical, it remains largely speculative. However, the capability for 3D scanning to quantify shape change, and for this to be linked to measured ground reaction forces and centre of gravity trajectory in a biomechanics laboratory, offers the potential to test the theory in an interdisciplinary manner.

In concluding this chapter, it is perhaps valuable to return to where we began. The diversity of the human form continues to captivate our interest, as we become increasingly aware of the threats to health and also of the specialisation of different sports. Clearly, quantifying adiposity is an important part of this metric, but one that requires the complementary information on shape, proportions and muscularity. The concept of rating these in an integrated system is robust, and although 3D scanning captures shape, it does not generate a somatotype rating. In addition it requires expensive specialised equipment and expertise for inter-pretation. However, the scope for using 3D scanned images as an alternative to the anthropometric and/or photoscopic somatotype is considerable, and may lead to renewed interest in this exciting area. This comes at a time when the scope for physique variation and specialisation is itself expanding. However, revisiting the original tenets of somatotype's early protagonists, it is hard to believe that it was not considered possible to have a more extreme physique than the original somatotype 'poles' of Sheldon as 7-1-1, 1-7-1 and 1-1-7. Extremes of physiques resulted from greater perturbation in the body's biologic processes have continually pushed back the frontiers of phenotypic variation since the 1940s. Endomorphy as high as 17 in an obese adolescent female (17-5-0.5), mesomorphy as high as 13 in a male bodybuilder (1-13-1) and ectomorphy as high as 13.5 in an anorexic female (1-1-13.5) have been reported (summarised in Olds, 2003). However, whether the boundaries of extreme phenotypic variation continue to expand in future is less certain. On one hand, advances in medicine may preserve life in those of extreme obesity or anorexia, and genetic manipulation may enable even greater muscle mass to be acquired. On the other hand, extremes in stature are being increasingly treated via hormonal and surgical interventions, hybridisation is blurring the ethnic-specific attributes associated with aboriginal peoples, and increasing globalisation and availability of mass media portraying idealised aspirational physiques, may decrease physique variability. Whether or not physique diversity has reached its zenith, science continues to demand reliable objective methods for quantifying human phenotypes, and we can anticipate this to be a vibrant area of future research.

References

Allen, B., Curless, B. & Popović, Z. (2003). The space of human body shapes: reconstruction and parameterization from range scans. *Association for Computing Machines Transactions on Graphics, 22*, 587–594.

Bandyopadhyay, A. (2007). Anthropometry and body composition in soccer and volleyball players in West Bengal, India. *Journal of Physiological Anthropology, 26*, 501–505.

Björntorp, P. (1988). Abdominal obesity and the development of noninsulin-dependent diabetes mellitus. *Diabetes Metabolism Research and Reviews, 4*, 615–622.

Bullen, A.K. & Hardy, H.L. (1946). Analysis of body build photographs of 175 college women. *American Journal of Physical Anthropology, 4*, 37–65.

Cameron, N. & Demerath, E.W. (2002). Critical periods in human growth and their relationship to diseases of aging. *Yearbook of Physical Anthropology, Supp. 35*, 159–184.

Carter, J.E.L. & Ackland, T.R. (2009). Somatotype in sport. In T.R. Ackland, B.C. Elliot and J. Bloomfield (Eds.) *Applied Anatomy and Biomechanics in Sport*, 2nd edition (pp. 47-66). Champaign, IL: Human Kinetics.

Carter, J.E.L. & Heath, B.H. (1990). *Somatotyping: Development and Applications*. Cambridge: Cambridge University Press.

Carter, J.E.L., Ackland, T.R., Kerr, D.A. & Stapff, A.B. (2005). Somatotype and size of elite female basketball players. *Journal of Sports Sciences, 23*, 1057–1063.

Damon, A. (1955). Physique and success in military flying. *American Journal of Physical Anthropology, 13*, 217–252.

Ducimetiere, P., Richard, J. & Cambian, F. (1986). The pattern of subcutaneous fat distribution in middle aged men and the risk of coronary heart disease. *International Journal of Obesity, 10*, 229–240.

Dupertuis, C.W. & Emanuel, I. (1956). *A Statistical Comparison of the Body Typing Methods of Hooton and Sheldon*. US Air Force, Wright Air Development Center. WADC Technical Report 56-366 (ASTIA Document AD 97205).

Duquet, W. & Carter, J.E.L. (2009). Somatotyping. In R. Eston and T. Reilly (Eds.) *Kinanthropometry and Exercise Physiology Laboratory Manual: Tests, Procedures and Data Vol. 1: Anthropometry*, 3rd edition (pp. 54–72). Abingdon: Routledge.

Garlie, T.N., Obusek, J.P., Corner, B.D. & Zambraski, E.J. (2010). Comparison of body fat estimates using 3D digital laser scans, direct manual anthropometry and DXA in men. *American Journal of Human Biology, 22*, 695–701.

Gaur, R., Maurya, M. & Kang, P.S. (2008). Sex, age and caste differences in somatotypes of Rajput and scheduled caste adolescents from the Sirmour District of Himachal Pradesh, India. *Anthropologischer Anzeiger, 66*, 81–97.

Ghosh, S. & Malik, S.L. (2010). Variations of body physique in Santhals: an Indian tribe. *Collegium Antropologicum, 34*, 467–472.

Goulding, M. (2010). *Somatotype: Calculation and Analysis* (CD-Rom software program). www.somatotype.org, South Australia: Sweat Technologies.

Heath, B.H. (1963). Need for modification of somatotype methodology. *American Journal of Physical Anthropology, 21*, 227–233.

Heath, B.H. & Carter, J.E.L. (1967). A modified somatotype method. *American Journal of Physical Anthropology, 27*, 57–74.

Holway, F.E. & Garavaglia, R. (2009). Kinanthropometry of Group I rugby players in Buenos Aires, Argentina. *Journal of Sports Sciences, 27*, 1211–1220.

Hooton, E.A. (1951). *Handbook of Body Types in the United States Army*. Cambridge, MA: Harvard University, Department of Anthropology.

Johnstone, A.M., Stewart, A.D., Benson, P.J., Kalafati, M., Rectenwald, L. and Horgan, G. (2008). Assessment of body image in obesity: development of a novel morphing technique. *Journal of Human Nutrition and Dietetics, 21*, 256–267.

Kahn, H.S., Austin, H., Williamson, D.F. & Arensberg, D. (1996). Simple anthropometric indices associated with ischemic heart disease. *Journal of Clinical Epidemiology, 49*, 1017–1024.

Keogh, J.W., Hume, P.A., Pearson, S.N. & Mellow, P. (2007). Anthropometric dimensions of male powerlifters of varying body mass. *Journal of Sports Sciences, 25*, 1365–1376.

Makgae, P.J., Monyeki, K.D., Brits, S.J., Kemper, H.C. & Mashita, J. (2007). Somatotype and blood pressure of rural South African children aged 6-13 years: Ellisras longitudinal growth and health study. *Annals of Human Biology, 34*, 240–251.

Mladenova, S., Nikolova, M., Andreenko, E. & Boyadjiev, D. (2010). Somatotypological characterization of Bulgarian children and adolescents (Smolyan region). *Collegium Antropologicum, 34*, 963–971.

Nevill, A.M., Stewart, A.D. & Olds, T. (2010). A simple explanation for the inverse association between height and weight in men. Letter, *American Journal of Clinical Nutrition, 92*, 1535.

Olds, T. (2003). Extreme physiques. In H. de Ridder & T. Olds (Eds.) *Kinanthropometry VII. Proceedings of the Seventh Scientific Conference of the International Society for the Advancement of Kinanthropometry, Brisbane, September 2000* (pp. 9–33). Potchefstroom: Potchefstroom University for Christian Higher Education.

Olds, T. & Honey, F. (2006). The use of 3D whole-body scanners in anthropometry. In M. Marfell-Jones, A. Stewart and T. Olds (Eds.) *Kinanthropometry IX. Proceedings of the 9th International Conference of the International Society for the Advancement of Kinanthropometry* (pp. 1–14). London: Routledge.

Parnell, R.W. (1954). Somatotyping by physical anthropometry. *American Journal of Physical Anthropology, 12*, 209–239.

Parnell, R.W. (1958). *Behavior and Physique.* London: Edward Arnold.

Pawlowski, B. (2001). The evolution of gluteal/femoral fat deposits and balance during pregnancy in bipedal Homo. *Current Anthropology, 42*, 572–574.

Preston, T.A. & Singh, M. (1972). Redintegrated somatotyping. *Ergonomics*, 15, 693-700.

Rebato, E., Jelenkovic, A. & Salces I. (2007). Heritability of the somatotype components in Biscay families. *HOMO - Journal of Comparative Human Biology, 58*, 199–210.

Saranga, S.P., Prista, A., Nhantumbo, L., Beunen, G., Rocha, J., Williams-Blangero, S. et al. (2008). Heritabilities of somatotype components in a population from rural Mozambique. *American Journal of Human Biology, 20*, 642–646.

Schranz, N., Tomkinson, G., Olds, T. & Daniell, N. (2010) Three-dimensional anthropometric analysis: differences between elite Australian rowers and the general population. *Journal of Sports Sciences, 28*, 459–469.

Sheldon, W.H., Stevens, S.S. & Tucker, W.B. (1940). *The Varieties of Human Physique.* New York: Harper and Brothers.

Stewart, A.D., Benson, P.J., Michanikou, E.G., Tsiota D. G. & Narli, M.K. (2003). Body image perception, satisfaction and somatotype in male and female athletes and non-athletes: results using a novel morphing technique. *Journal of Sports Sciences, 21*, 815–823.

Stewart, A.D., Giles, K., Johnstone, A.M. & Benson, P. J. (2008). Physique relationships in body dissatisfaction. In M. Marfell-Jones and T. Olds (Eds.) *Kinanthropometry X. Proceedings of the 10th International Society for the Advancement of Kinanthropometry Conference* (pp. 231–241). London: Routledge.

Stewart, A.D., Klein, S., Young, J., Simpson, S., Lee, A.J., Harrild, K. et al. (2012). Body image, shape, and volumetric assessments using 3D whole body laser scanning and 2D digital photography in females with a diagnosed eating disorder: Preliminary novel findings. *British Journal of Psychology*, online early view DOI:10.1111/j.2044-8295.2011.02063.x.

Stewart, A.D., Marfell-Jones, M., Olds, T. & de Ridder, H. (2011). *International Standards for Anthropometric Assessment*. Potchefstroom: ISAK.

Stewart, A.D. Nevill, A.M., Stephen R. & Young, J. (2010). Waist size and shape assessed by 3D photonic scanning. *International Journal of Body Composition Research, 8*, 123–130.

Tanner, J.M. (1964). *The Physique of the Olympic Athlete*. London: George Allen and Unwin Ltd.

Tucker, W.B. & Lessa, W.A. (1940). Man: a constitutional investigation. *The Quarterly Review of Biology, 15*, 411–455.

Voracek, M. &Fisher, M.L. (2002). Shapely centrefolds? Temporal change in body measures: trend analysis. *British Medical Journal, 325*, 1447–1448.

Wang, J., Gallagher, D., Thornton, J.C., Yu, W., Horlick, M. & Pi-Sunyer, F.X. (2006). Validation of a 3-dimensional photonic scanner for the measurement of body volumes, dimensions, and percentage body fat. *American Journal of Clinical Nutrition, 83*, 809–816.

Wang, J., Thornton, J.C., Bari, S., Williamson, B., Gallagher, D., Heymsfield, S.B. et al. (2003). Comparisons of waist circumferences measured at 4 sites *American Journal of Clinical Nutrition, 77*, 379–384.

Wells, J.C.K., Cole, T.J. & Treleaven, P. (2008a). Age-variability in body shape associated with excess weight: the UK national sizing survey. *Obesity, 16*, 435–441.

Wells, J.C.K., Cole, T.J., Bruner, D. & Treleaven, P. (2008b). Body shape in American and British adults: between-country and inter-ethnic comparisons. *International Journal of Obesity, 32*, 152–159.

Wells, J.C.K., Treleaven, P. & Cole, T.J. (2007). BMI compared with 3-dimensional body shape: the UK national sizing survey. *American Journal of Clinical Nutrition, 85*, 419–425.

5

MUSCLE TISSUE

Laura Sutton

This chapter will cover:

5.1   Muscle anatomy and physiology
5.2   Relevance to physical activity, lifestyle and health
5.3   Responses to exercise training
5.4   Estimation of muscle mass *in vivo*

5.1 Muscle anatomy and physiology

Muscles have been described as 'among the most intricate machines on the planet' (Germann & Stanfield, 2002, p.334). In this first section, an overview of the structure and function of muscle tissue will be provided; for a more comprehensive exposition, the reader is directed to any dedicated anatomy and physiology text.

5.1.1 Definition and types of tissue

Muscle tissue is a contractile tissue made up of muscle cells, connective tissue and extracellular materials. The word muscle originates from the Latin term *musculus*, meaning 'small mouse' – a reference to the appearance of certain muscles, for example the biceps brachii, when undergoing contraction. The role of muscle tissue is to produce force and effect bodily movement. The muscle cells within the tissue have contractile properties and the ability to conduct electrical impulses, making movement possible. The cells themselves contain contractile proteins, details of which are given in Section 5.1.3.

According to young, healthy adult reference values developed by Dr Albert Behnke, the average proportion of body mass made up of muscle tissue is estimated at 44.8 per cent in men and 36.0 per cent in women (McArdle, Katch

& Katch, 2009). There are three distinct types of muscle tissue: cardiac, skeletal and smooth (Table 5.1). The majority of the body's muscle mass is composed of skeletal muscle, which is the main component of the fat-free mass. In keeping with the scope of the chapter, subsequent text will refer specifically to skeletal muscle tissue.

TABLE 5.1 Different types of muscle tissue

Tissue	Description	Example location
Skeletal	Also known as voluntary muscle tissue, skeletal muscle tissue is so named due to being affixed to the skeleton by tendons. The tissue is striated, meaning it has a striped appearance, due to the arrangement of filaments within the myofibrils	Biceps brachii
Smooth	Smooth muscle tissue may be referred to as involuntary muscle tissue, due to its action not being under conscious control. It is described as smooth due to its lack of visible striations. Smooth muscles are located in the walls of hollow structures, such as blood vessels and internal organs	Intestinal wall
Cardiac	A specialised tissue found only in the heart, cardiac muscle tissue is closer in structure to skeletal muscle, yet like smooth muscle is under involuntary control	Heart muscle

5.1.2 Muscle fibre types

There is some inconsistency in the literature as to the number and categories of different types of muscle fibre. There are various classification schemes, for example, distinction according to the myosin heavy chain (MHC) isoform (fibre types I, IIA, IIX and IIB), isometric contraction time (slow-twitch and fast-twitch fibres) and fatigue properties (fast-fatiguable, fast-fatigue resistant and slow-fatigue resistant fibres). Although the different methods of delineation should not be considered equivalent, they are generally correlated, and the main groupings are listed below, using the myosin profile as the primary categorisation scheme:

Type I – slow oxidative, or 'slow twitch' fibres. Type I fibres are capillary-dense and myoglobin-rich. Whilst relatively slow to contract, they are fatigue-resistant. They are required for aerobic activity such as maintaining posture and sustained physical activity, for example endurance sports.

Type IIA – fast oxidative or 'fast twitch A' fibres, so named for their ability to contract rapidly, but maintain oxidative processes. They are used during both aerobic and anaerobic activities.

Type IIB – fast glycolytic or 'fast twitch B' fibres, meaning they contain a high amount of glycogen, but lower amounts of myoglobin and fewer mitochondria and capillaries than type IIA fibres. They produce energy rapidly, yet fatigue quickly. They are required for explosive activity, for example sprinting.

More recently, a fourth main fibre type was identified: the fast-twitch fibre IID, IIX or IID(X). Type IID fibres have properties in between those of type IIA and IIB fibres. Owing to their similarity to type IIB fibres, IID fibres were previously included in this category; refined methodology now allows delineation of the two types. Skeletal muscle fibres are generally categorised into two, three or four discrete groups in this manner for the sake of simplicity, but in actual fact they are better defined according to a continuum. Muscle fibres may fall at some point along a spectrum ranging from type I to type IIB, and may be a 'pure' fibre (single MHC isoform), such as the groups described above, or a hybrid (≥ 2 MHC isoforms), for example, a type I/IIA fibre (Pette & Staron, 2001). The fibres innervated by a given motor neuron will all be of the same type.

Skeletal muscles are composed of a mixture of fibre types, and muscle groups will have differing optimal compositions depending on their primary purpose. The reader is referred to Section 5.3.3 for a discussion of the effects of training on muscle fibre composition.

5.1.3 Muscular contraction

The force-generating part of the muscle is composed of bundles of muscle cells (fibres), connective tissue, nerves and blood vessels. Muscle cells have multiple nuclei and each fibre contains bundles of protein filaments called myofibrils. Myofibrils in turn contain thin and thick filaments – proteins which are called actin and myosin – which are joined by cross-bridges located at the myosin head. One complete unit is referred to as a sarcomere. An illustration of the muscle fibres is provided in Figure 5.1.

A mechanism of muscle contraction referred to as the 'sliding filament theory', proposed simultaneously by H. Huxley & Hanson (1954) and A. Huxley & Niedergerke (1954), provides the accepted model of muscular contraction. The researchers noted that muscle filaments themselves do not contract, but slide past one another, to bring about the observed shortening of sarcomeres. Whilst the sliding filament theory was not instantly widely accepted, further articles were published in the 1950s and 1970s in which a 'cross-bridge cycle' was described, explaining the mechanism behind the sliding filament theory and leading to its general acceptance. The cross-bridge cycle is illustrated in Figure 5.2.

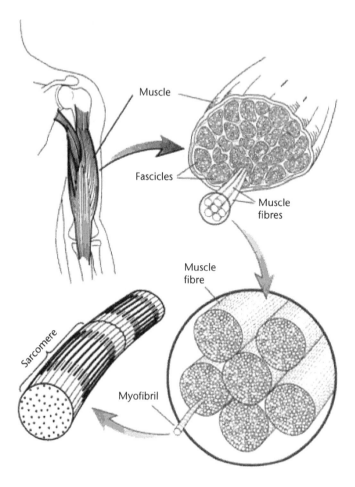

FIGURE 5.1 Structural hierarchy of skeletal muscle (source: Lieber (2002). *Skeletal Muscle Structure, Function and Plasticity: The Physiological Basis of Rehabilitation.* Copyright © 2002 Lippincott Williams & Wilkins).

Definition of terms (in descending order of magnitude):

- **Muscle fibre** – a muscle cell, made up of myofibrils
- **Myofibril** – an aggregation of parallel protein filaments forming contractile units
- **Sarcomere** – one contractile unit within the myofibril
- **Filaments** – thick and thin filaments, made up of the proteins myosin and actin, respectively
- **Thin filaments** – in addition to actin, the thin filaments contain troponin and tropomyosin, proteins which regulate muscle contraction

The cross-bridge cycle is powered by the breakdown of adenosine triphosphate (ATP) molecules, the main direct source of energy for cellular activity, by the enzyme myosin ATPase. As shown in Figure 5.2, the myosin head begins detached from the thin filament, the head is then 'cocked', using energy from the hydrolysis of ATP, and binds to the actin. What follows is termed a 'power stroke', which is a rowing motion during which the myosin pulls the actin towards the centre of the sarcomere, releasing stored energy. The myosin and actin remain bound in a state of 'rigour', until unbinding is triggered by a new ATP molecule and the cycle is repeated. Each myosin head completes around five cycles per second during contraction, and each filament has several hundred heads, allowing fibres to contract very rapidly (Germann & Stanfield, 2002).

Skeletal muscle contractions are controlled by the nervous system. Nerve cells called motor neurons are connected to muscle fibres via neuromuscular junctions. Each fibre is served by just one motor neuron. The motor neuron transmits an impulse, triggering the release of the neurotransmitter acetylcholine, which travels across the neuromuscular junction. Its binding at the muscle cell triggers an 'action potential' which, through the release of calcium ions, stimulates the cross-bridge cycle, enabling contraction. When a motor neuron ceases its input, the associated muscle fibre will stop contracting.

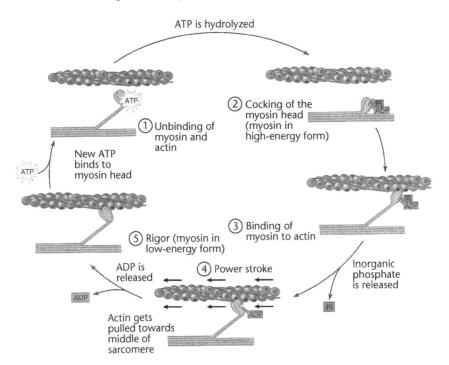

FIGURE 5.2 The cross-bridge cycle (source: Germann & Stanfield (2008). *Principles of Human Physiology* (3rd edition) © 2008. Reprinted by permission of Pearson Education, Inc., Upper Saddle River, NJ).

The term 'muscle contraction' implies a shortening of the muscle, but in fact a muscle may shorten, lengthen or maintain its length whilst its fibres undergo contraction. A shortening of muscle length under tension is referred to as *concentric* contraction. Extension of a muscle under tension is referred to as *eccentric* contraction. An *isometric* contraction is one in which force is generated without a concurrent change in muscle length or joint angle. Whilst colloquially used in the fitness industry to denote a 'lean' physique, from a physiological perspective the term 'muscle tone' actually describes a continuous, partial state of contraction in a muscle. Muscle tone, or 'tonus', produces a state of physical readiness and helps maintain balance and posture.

5.1.4 Hypertrophy and atrophy

Muscle growth is termed hypertrophy and muscle loss is referred to as atrophy. An additional process (not covered in detail in the present chapter) is hyperplasia, which refers to the generation of new muscle cells. Pathways regulating hypertrophy and atrophy are influenced by a number of factors including physical activity and loading, nutrient availability and various growth factors.

Natural hypertrophy occurs during growth, but muscular hypertrophy may also be brought about by physical training. Hypertrophy may be classified as sarcoplasmic or myofibrillar. Sarcoplasmic hypertrophy, as the name suggests, involves growth of the sarcoplasm, which is the specific name for the cytoplasm (jelly-like cellular material) in skeletal muscle fibres. Fibres increase in volume due to the expansion of the sarcoplasm and growth of non-contractile proteins. Conversely, myofibrillar hypertrophy involves the synthesis of contractile proteins, leading to an increase in filament density.

Colloquially referred to as muscle 'wasting', muscular atrophy is characterised by a loss of muscle mass. A reduction in protein content occurs when the rate of degradation exceeds that of synthesis, and muscle cells decrease in size and number. Atrophy may occur for various reasons, for example as a result of illness, ageing, starvation or physical inactivity. During illness, atrophy may occur as a direct consequence of disease, or indirectly through prolonged bed-rest. It is associated with many chronic conditions, such as heart disease, cancer and disability (see Chapter 9). Further causes of atrophy include extreme conditions, such as weightlessness (see Reilly & Waterhouse, 2005, for further detail).

5.2 Relevance to physical activity, lifestyle and health

The muscular system has many roles essential to normal physiological functioning. Without the muscular system, processes essential to life, such as blood circulation, respiration and digestion, would not be possible. Muscles allow locomotion, maintain posture, stabilise joints and act as 'shock absorbers', reducing the risk of injury to the body. Heat generation is another important role, aiding the regulation of body temperature.

5.2.1 Muscle mass and energy expenditure

The basal metabolic rate (BMR) is rate at which energy is expended in order to maintain vital functions when the body is in a post-absorptive, resting state in a thermoneutral environment. In healthy populations there is a positive correlation between muscle mass and BMR meaning that, in general, the greater the muscle mass, the greater the amount of energy expended at rest. Muscle tissue is metabolically more active than many other tissues, for example bone and adipose tissue, meaning that, for a given quantity, muscle tissue will require more energy when in a resting state. However, it should be noted that the majority of basal energy expenditure is attributable to the body's vital organs.

Total energy expenditure (TEE) is the average overall amount of energy expended, usually estimated over a typical 24-hour period. On a basic level, TEE accounts for basal energy expenditure, energy expended during physical activity and the thermic effect of feeding. Further energy requirements may arise, for example the additional energy demands of pregnancy or childhood growth. Generally, after accounting for BMR, physical activity contributes the most to TEE. Energy expenditure is increased during exercise and during the post-exercise recovery period, with the type and intensity of exercise determining the magnitude of the response. An overview of the chronic effects of training and different exercise modalities on the muscle compartment is provided in Section 5.3.

5.2.2 Dietary requirements

The amino acids found in dietary protein sources are essential for the maintenance of muscle mass and are often referred to as the 'building blocks' of body proteins. The majority of the body's protein is located within skeletal muscle tissue. Muscle tissue undergoes protein turnover, where protein is broken down by a process called degradation and replaced through protein synthesis. The availability of amino acids in the body is a key regulator of protein synthesis.

In the human body, 20 different amino acids are used to create proteins, eight of which are termed 'essential amino acids' as they cannot be synthesised in the body and, therefore, must be provided by dietary intake. Wolfe (2002) found a constant amino acid intake to stimulate protein synthesis in a dose-dependent manner until concentrations are approximately doubled, with higher doses having no additional effect, and low levels inhibiting protein synthesis.

Protein is required for many vital processes, and if there is insufficient protein in the diet, the body will metabolise protein stored in the muscles. Insufficient materials for protein synthesis lead to an imbalance in protein turnover, and the excess degradation leads to muscular atrophy. Other symptoms of insufficient protein/amino acid intake include fatigue, irritability and decreased appetite. Extreme cases of protein deficiency, such as those observed in developing countries, often result in retarded growth and mental development, oedema, disease and, in some cases, death.

There has been much debate over dietary protein and associated amino acid and nitrogen requirements. The required intake will be dictated by many factors, including but not limited to age, gender, body size and composition, physical activity, physiological state and overall energy requirements. The current recommended safe daily protein intake for healthy adults is around $0.83\,g.kg^{-1}$ (WHO, 2007). Maintaining an increased muscle mass increases nutritional requirements, and many athletes supplement their dietary intake with nutritional supplements such as protein-rich drinks and bars, and amino acid drinks or tablets. Despite not demonstrating a large muscle mass, endurance athletes also have increased protein requirements, as training stimulates the protein turnover process and, during long-duration endurance activities, protein may be broken down to provide fuel. Carbohydrates and fats are also important, as muscle contractions are predominantly powered by the oxidation of these substrates.

5.2.3 Gender differences

As noted earlier, the relative amounts of muscle mass differ between men and women (reference man has almost 10 per cent more of his overall body mass made up of muscle mass). Men generally have greater regional and total skeletal muscle mass. As would be expected, differences in strength and power tend to be evident between men and women. Women generally generate less force, and have a lower ratio of upper-to-lower-body strength. When considering strength relative to total body mass, as opposed to absolute values, men may still be stronger than women, more notably so in the upper body. Aside from differences in average height and the proportion of body mass comprised of fat-free mass, women generally have a smaller muscle fibre cross-sectional area than men, which may contribute to their overall lower strength. Gender differences may be notable during the ageing process, as the menopause has been associated with a greater loss of muscle mass in women. Gender differences in muscle mass, strength and power are evident in both trained and untrained populations.

Fleck & Kraemer (2004) reported that resistance training is at least as, if not more, beneficial for women than men. Despite a common fear that resistance training will render a woman too 'bulky', their review of the literature showed that relative peak oxygen consumption may increase, adaptations are evident in the muscle compartment without excessive hypertrophy, and favourable changes are usually evident in overall body composition. (See Section 5.3.1 for an exploration of the physiological responses to resistance training.)

5.2.4 Age-related changes in muscle mass

Changes in body composition brought about by changes to the muscle compartment impact upon components of physical fitness, metabolism and health. Muscle strength is important for force production and injury prevention. The overall strength of a muscle depends upon the number of fibres, the physiological cross-sectional area (the area of a slice that would allow a view of most, if not all, the fibres in a muscle) and optimal muscle fibre recruitment. Given the relationship between force and mass/area, muscular atrophy usually leads to a decrease in muscle strength. Loss of strength may in turn increase the risk of injury and is generally associated with a lower quality of life, particularly in older persons.

The age-related loss of muscle mass and strength is termed 'sarcopenia', from the Greek meaning 'poverty of flesh'. It is caused both by the ageing process and by age-associated reductions in physical activity. Initial muscle atrophy is slow, but increases with advancing age. Muscle fibre composition tends to undergo alteration, with a loss of type II fibres resulting in a greater proportion of type I fibres. Sarcopenia affects both men and women and is an important consideration, given the potential for increased physical impairment. The risk of falling is greater, and falls may lead to fracture and hospitalisation.

Furthermore, the reduction in metabolically active tissue is associated with a reduction in metabolism. If dietary intake is not adjusted accordingly, further unfavourable changes in body composition may occur, for example, an increase in adiposity. In addition, lower metabolic heat production reduces the ability of the body to cope in cold conditions. Whilst it becomes more difficult to accrue muscle mass with age, it is not impossible, and at the very least, age-related decreases in mass and function may be slowed with regular exercise.

5.3 Responses to exercise training

5.3.1 Strength stimuli

Strength, or resistance, training encompasses exercises in which muscles are required to contract against resistance provided by external, opposing forces. This training style is sometimes referred to as weight training but, whilst weight training generally refers to the use of free weights, such as dumbbells and barbells, and weight training machines, the term resistance training is broader, encompassing other methods of training such as plyometrics.

Resistance training is generally used to increase muscle force-generating capacity, elicit a hypertrophic response or enhance muscular endurance. Such training requires a high rate of anaerobic energy production. Different training modalities may be employed, depending on the purpose of the training. Examples of different types of resistance training include:

- *Isotonic training* – consists of concentric-eccentric contractions; resistance may be constant or variable across the range of movement. *Eccentric-only* exercises take advantage of the fact that greater loads may be lowered than lifted to utilise a greater resistance than may be managed in concentric-eccentric contractions.
- *Isometric training* – makes use of isometric contractions to increase static strength. A force may be applied to an immovable object or static resistance applied against an external force.

- *Isokinetic training* – uses specialised equipment that continually adjusts the resistance to create a constant rate of contraction. Isokinetic exercises incorporate isotonic and isometric elements.

It is generally accepted that resistance training causes microtrauma in the muscle fibres, particularly during eccentric muscle action. Protein filaments are broken down during resistance exercise (catabolism); they are then restored during the subsequent recovery period (anabolism). It is thought that the body over-compensates for the training-induced damage, leading to a bolstered anabolic phase (supercompensation), resulting in muscular hypertrophy. The brief, repeated, submaximal or maximal efforts associated with resistance training place great emphasis on the type II muscle fibres. Whilst much of the associated increase in muscle size may be attributed to the hypertrophy of type II fibres, it has been argued that hyperplasia also takes place in response to strength training. However, this is likely to account for a small proportion of muscle growth. The discomfort experienced as a result of microtrauma, typically a day or two after exercise, is termed 'delayed onset muscle soreness' (DOMS). The soreness is distinct from that experienced during injury and tends to be greater following changes to an exercise programme such as the introduction of a new exercise or an increase in training intensity.

The amount of force a muscle may generate is related to its cross-sectional area, which is determined by the number of muscle fibres and the fibre cross-sectional area. Both sarcoplasmic and myofibrillar hypertrophy may occur in response to training. Muscular hypertrophy results in an increased capacity for force production due to the increase in contractile elements. Thus, increases in muscle strength are generally associated with hypertrophy, particularly myofibrillar hypertrophy. However, there are other factors in addition to hypertrophy that may increase force generation. Neural adaptations to training may produce increases in strength, as the nervous system improves in its ability to recruit the appropriate muscles. The greater the activation of agonistic muscles and the more efficient the recruitment pattern for a given movement, the greater the force that may be generated. A high proportion of the initial increases in strength resulting from resistance training will occur as a result of neural adaptations.

Specific details of neuromuscular physiology, tendon biomechanics and further adaptations to strength training are beyond the scope of this book. Instead, readers are referred to Cardinale, Newton & Nosaka (2011) for a recent comprehensive text. Individuals engaging in resistance training will frequently seek the optimal training modality, combination of sets and repetitions, overall training volume and rest time; however, it should be borne in mind that what is optimal for one individual may not be so for another. For example, optimal set/rep combinations will depend upon many factors, including the specific purpose of the training, the targeted muscle groups and the individual's level of experience, amongst others. For a comprehensive overview of resistance training programme design the reader is directed to the work of Fleck & Kraemer (2004).

Muscle adaptations to sprint training are similar to those observed with resistance training. Muscle cross-sectional area increases as a result of sarcoplasmic and myofibrillar hypertrophy. The anaerobic nature of sprint training places emphasis on the type IIA muscle fibres, and neural adaptations improve their recruitment. Mitochondrial enzyme activity also increases, allowing faster recovery between bouts and following training sessions.

There is broad symmetry in the body as a whole, although some asymmetry may occur to an extent naturally in the upper limbs due to the use of the dominant limb for a range of tasks. (It is customary to make anthropometric measurements on the right-hand side of the body as, for the majority of individuals, it is the dominant side.) For most individuals, asymmetry is not measurable in the lower limbs, and any differences tend to fall within measurement error in anthropometry and relate to pixel size and regional boundaries in dual X-ray absorptiometry (DXA). However, sports-specific training can induce notable asymmetry with certain repetitive movements, particularly in unilateral activities such as fencing and racquet sports. For example, Stewart (unpublished data) found an athlete competing in fencing to demonstrate a 15 per cent and 8 per cent difference between dominant and non-dominant sides in arm and leg fat-free soft-tissue mass, and a badminton athlete to show a 24 per cent and 2 per cent difference between sides in arm and leg fat-free soft-tissue mass, respectively. Such asymmetry may predispose athletes to injury, and training for the non-dominant side may assist in injury prevention.

5.3.2 Endurance stimuli

Whilst there are different forms of endurance, for example aerobic, anaerobic and local muscular strength endurance, the term endurance training is generally used to refer to exercise programmes that predominantly target the aerobic energy system. Endurance exercise may be continuous in nature, known as 'steady state' exercise, or may incorporate interval training. Common examples of activities include running, swimming and cycling.

Muscular responses to endurance training include increased capillarisation, allowing greater oxygen delivery and heat dissipation, and increased mitochondrial density in the muscle fibres predominantly recruited during exercise, increasing their oxidative capacity. Glucose uptake is improved, as is the ability to store glucose and fat in the muscle. Lipolysis, which is the breakdown of fat, is enhanced, facilitating the use of fat as an energy source. Aerobic enzymes are also increased, improving the efficiency of the energy production process.

In addition to skeletal muscle-specific adaptations, adaptations to endurance training occur in other body systems, including the cardiovascular and nervous systems. Biochemical and metabolic adaptations are also effected. The chronic responses to endurance training lead to improvements in maximal oxygen uptake, which is the maximum capacity for the transport and use of oxygen during exercise, and the anaerobic or lactate threshold, which is the point at which lactic acid begins to accumulate in the blood. Endurance-trained individuals also tend to be more efficient and demonstrate greater exercise economy than their untrained counterparts, expending less energy at a given workload. In many cases, shifts in body composition are also evident, with endurance training associated with a reduction in adipose tissue and total body mass.

5.3.3 Changes in fibre composition

Skeletal muscle tissue demonstrates plasticity and, whilst muscle phenotype is predominantly determined by genetic factors, it may also adapt in response to exercise stimuli and other factors, such as altered motorneuron activity, hormonal profiles and ageing. It has been suggested that the MHC isoforms defining the muscle fibre type transition from slow to fast or vice versa in a sequential manner according to the continuum described in Section 5.1.2. The most common transition resulting from exercise training is a IIB-IIA shift (Pette & Staron, 2001). However, the exact mechanisms responsible have yet to be fully determined. Exercise training will not change individual type I fibres to type II fibres, or vice versa, but preferential hypertrophy of a given fibre type can alter the proportion of fibre types within a muscle, as increases in fibre cross-sectional area result in the fibre type accounting for a greater proportion of the muscle.

In a review of resistance training studies, Fry (2004) reported recurring evidence of the IIB-IIA shift following high intensity training. The finding is surprising as, given the faster contraction, it may be assumed that IIB fibres would be preferential for heavy resistance exercise. However, it has been hypothesised that IIB fibres are not as frequently used as they are more difficult to recruit, thus making type IIA the preferred fibre type. Long-term sprint training also induces a shift towards IIA fibres. Type I fibres have not been found to convert to type II properties as a result of strength training, but decrease in proportion as type II fibres undergo hypertrophy.

The conversion of type IIB fibres is also possible through endurance training. Whilst submaximal exercise involves high type I recruitment, maximal exertion involves higher recruitment of type IIA fibres, promoting a IIB-IIA shift. The relative proportion of type I fibres in targeted muscles may increase as the fibre area increases. Endurance-trained athletes tend to have more type I muscle fibres than untrained counterparts, although it is uncertain to what extent this finding is due to athlete self-selection, as individuals with a higher oxidative capacity may naturally tend towards more endurance-based activities.

5.3.4 The effects of overtraining

The overtraining syndrome occurs when training volume is excessive and/or insufficient time is allowed for post-training recovery. Whilst there are many physiological manifestations of overtraining, those pertaining to the muscle compartment include structural, biochemical and neuromuscular alterations which cause muscle damage, soreness, fatigue and an increased risk of injury.

Muscular atrophy may occur as protein synthesis is decreased and degradation increased, resulting in the destruction of myofibrils, and reduction of satellite cells, which play an integral role in the growth and repair of muscle tissue. Detrimental effects on body composition may be noted, as the catabolism of muscle tissue can reduce overall muscle mass and total body weight. The musculoskeletal system is also affected by an increased risk of overuse injuries such as stress fractures and tendonitis.

Changes at the neuromuscular junction may have adverse effects on muscle contraction and relaxation. Muscle glycogen concentration is often reduced due to insufficient recovery between intense training bouts. However, overtraining symptoms may still be evident in the presence of maintained energy stores. As a result of the detrimental physiological adaptations, muscular strength and endurance commonly decrease, and the ability to perform at a high intensity is reduced.

5.3.5 The effects of detraining

When exercise training is reduced significantly or stopped entirely, the physical adaptations brought about by training are gradually lost. The reduction in physical activity may result from a conscious decision or be brought about by injury or illness. A regression towards the pre-training state occurs. The main factors affecting the rate at which changes such as muscular atrophy occur include the individual's body composition and level of training prior to cessation, and the extent of the reduction in activity, with greater declines evident in more highly-trained athletes and a greater reduction in training load associated with faster detraining. Age is also an influential factor, with a faster decline upon training cessation expected in older persons, particularly post-menopausal women.

The size of the skeletal muscle fibres and the number of satellite cells, both of which increase in response to training stimuli, will eventually return to pre-training values. The associated loss of muscle mass is accompanied by a decreased capacity for force generation. Reductions in strength and power are brought about by both the reduction in fibre cross-sectional area and a reduction in fibre recruitment. Muscular endurance and flexibility are reduced with atrophy. Aerobic performance will also suffer following periods of detraining, as the number of capillaries may decrease, reducing oxygen uptake by muscle cells. Glycogen stores in the muscle also tend to decrease.

Muscle fibre conversions brought about by long-term training may be reversed, returning the fibre properties to pre-training status. The characteristics of type II fibres may shift back from IIA characteristics to those of type IIB. The training-induced hypertrophy of muscle fibres specific to the exercise demands is also reversed, shifting the relative proportions back towards pre-training composition. The rate and extent of any detraining-related adaptations can be attenuated if some level of activity is maintained.

In the event of injury or immobilisation to one limb or one side of the body, the affected area may undergo the effects of detraining. However, it has been shown that resistance training the corresponding uninjured limbs may attenuate the loss of strength and size in the muscles of inactive limbs through a neurological process termed 'cross-education'. The exact underlying mechanisms have yet to be determined, but the effect can be seen in men and women of different ages and, whilst cross-education is not restricted to particular muscle groups, the effect is specific to the contra-lateral corresponding muscle (Lee & Carroll, 2007).

5.4 Estimation of muscle mass *in vivo*

The ability to estimate muscle mass *in vivo* has its uses in a number of applied settings. In the clinical setting, estimations of muscle mass may contribute to the monitoring of childhood growth and development, malnutrition and disease progression. Measurements may be used to determine the effects of interventions designed to improve body composition and health outcomes. In a sporting context, the effects of dietary and training interventions on the muscle compartment may be monitored, along with any associated changes in performance. Muscle mass may also be used to normalise physiological parameters in research settings. As is common in applied body composition analysis, a number of methods exist, the choice of which may be determined by the purpose of assessment and the equipment, personnel and finances available.

5.4.1 Anthropometric estimation of muscle mass

In 1921, anthropologist Jindrich Matiegka published equations for the prediction of tissue mass from body surface measurements, in a bid to estimate so-called 'physical efficiency'. Estimations of muscle mass (M) were as follows:

$$M = k_3 \times r^2 \times L$$
$$M = k_4 \times c^2 \times L$$

The coefficients 'k_3' and 'k_4' were described as assumed coefficients to be determined by cadaver analysis. The quantities 'r' and 'c' represent the average radius and average circumference of the extremities corrected for skin and subcutaneous adipose tissue thickness, resulting in what Matiegka termed the 'muscular column'. Average values are obtained by calculating the mean of the circumferences from the following anatomic sites: the (flexed) biceps, the mid-thigh, and the forearm and calf at maximum girth. The quantity 'L' represents the stature; measurements of stature and circumference are taken in centimetres.

Matiegka's formulae were revised by Drinkwater, Martin, Ross & Clarys in 1986. Using the first of his proposed formulae for the estimation of muscle mass, Matiegka provided an estimate for k_3 of 6.5. Using data from 13 cadavers, Drinkwater and colleagues re-estimated the coefficient to be 7.11. In a further cadaver study, Martin, Spenst, Drinkwater & Clarys (1990) revised the work of Matiegka, providing the following updated formula:

$$M = L \times (0.0553 \times CTG^2 + 0.0987 \times FG^2 + 0.0331 \times CCG^2) - 2445$$

where CTG is the thigh circumference corrected for the anterior thigh skinfold thickness, FG is the uncorrected forearm circumference and CCG is the calf circumference corrected for the medial calf skinfold thickness; skinfold thicknesses are measured in centimetres. Note that the model of Martin et al. used the skinfold multiplied by π in order to produce corrected girths in a circular concentric model.

Regional muscle mass or area may be assessed by girth measurement, corrected for skin and adipose tissue thickness by way of skinfold caliper measurement. The most common site for measurement is the upper arm. Gurney & Jelliffe (1973) provided nomograms for the estimation of muscle cross-sectional area from arm circumference. Heymsfield, McManus, Smith, Stevens & Nixon (1982) later revised equations of Jelliffe, providing gender-specific equations for the estimation of muscle area corrected for bone area in addition to adipose tissue. Regional muscle mass is taken to be proportional to overall skeletal muscle mass. As with all anthropometric techniques for assessing body composition, the method is subject to a number of assumptions and potential sources of error, and tends to lose accuracy the greater the adiposity of the individual. However, the low cost and simplicity and speed of measurement make the anthropometric estimation of muscle area a useful tool in many field-based settings.

5.4.2 Metabolic techniques

The endogenous excretion of muscle metabolites may be used to estimate muscle mass and metabolism, based on assumptions such as the metabolites being specific to muscle tissue and having relatively constant rates of turnover. Creatinine excretion is proportional to the amount of creatine stored in the body, the majority of which may be found in muscle tissue; therefore the measurement of creatinine provides an indirect measure of total muscle mass. Urinary 3-methylhistidine (3-MH) excretion is also used as a predictor of muscle mass, as the amino acid 3-MH is found predominantly in muscle tissue. Both metabolites are released during muscle protein breakdown, and may be measured through urinary analysis.

Laboratory-based techniques such as muscle metabolite testing tend to produce more valid and reliable results than more crude assessments. However, such tests have limitations, for example, the need for a meat-free diet to be consumed prior to testing in order to limit intake of the metabolite from dietary sources. Expensive assay equipment is required, and tests tend to require specific timing and a longer duration than alternative methods of assessment. Age may need to be taken into consideration, as changes in body composition with ageing may mean metabolite concentration and excretion are not always constant. Gender differences may need to be considered also.

5.4.3 Nuclear techniques

Potassium is a mineral and electrolyte which forms an important constituent of muscle tissue. The concentration of potassium in the fat-free mass has been estimated at around 2.5–2.7 g/kg fat-free mass from cadaver analyses, and is considered constant. As mentioned in Chapter 2, Potassium-40 (K^{40}) is a radioactive isotope of potassium naturally occurring in the human body. It emits gamma rays, therefore gamma ray spectroscopy may be used to 'count' the potassium in the body. Fat-free mass can be predicted from estimations of total-body potassium by external K^{40} counting. However, K^{40} alone tends to remain an indicator of fat-free mass or body cell mass rather than actual muscle mass. It is limited in its use as an estimator of total muscle mass as K^{40} is present in other body tissues.

Protein contains ~16 per cent nitrogen and nearly all of the nitrogen in the body may be found in protein, meaning estimations of total-body nitrogen may be converted to estimations of total-body protein. By combining measurements of total-body potassium and nitrogen, the total-body protein mass may be divided into muscle and non-muscle compartments based on assumed values, allowing for an estimation of total muscle mass. Both total-body nitrogen and potassium may be measured using *in vivo* neutron activation analysis. Nuclear techniques are often used as reference methods, given their high precision and the ability to quantify multiple elements. However, this approach is costly, requires specialist equipment, involves radiation exposure, and is often not practical for use.

5.4.4 Radiographic techniques

Technological advances now allow for estimation of muscle mass by medical imaging techniques such as magnetic resonance imaging (MRI) and computed tomography (CT). These methods provide *in vivo* 'gold standard' techniques for the estimation of mass, cross-sectional area and volume. Such measures of muscle tissue are useful indicators of disease and conditions such as sarcopenia. Both regional and total-body analyses are possible. Examples of MRI images, showing an untrained and a resistance-trained individual, are provided in Figure 5.3; the tissue appearing dark grey in colour is the muscle tissue. However, due to high cost and limited availability, the use of MRI and CT scanning is mainly restricted to medical settings. In addition, exposure to ionising radiation precludes the routine use of CT scanning.

The fat-free soft-tissue mass computed by DXA is frequently used as a surrogate measure of muscle mass. As skeletal muscle accounts for the largest proportion of the fat-free soft-tissue compartment, the two measures are highly correlated. Although the technique does not provide a direct assessment of muscle mass, DXA provides a cheaper and faster alternative to MRI and CT, and exposes the participant to much less radiation than CT scanning. An example of a whole-body DXA image is provided in Figure 5.4; the muscle tissue appears light grey in colour.

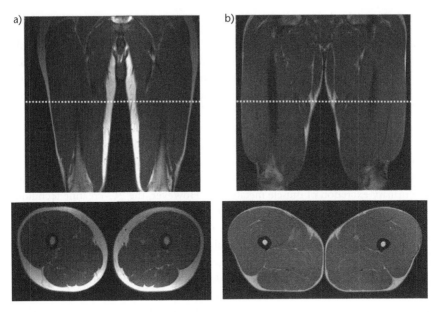

FIGURE 5.3 Coronal and axial MRI images of the thigh of resistance trained (R) and untrained (L) men (source: D'Antona et al. (2006). *Journal of Physiology*, 570, 611–627. Reprinted with permission of John Wiley & Sons, Inc.).

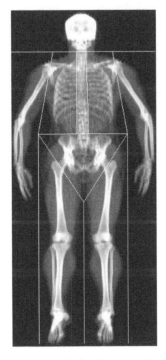

FIGURE 5.4 Whole-body DXA image of a healthy man (image © Laura Sutton).

5.4.5 Total-body water

Measurements of total-body water are often used to estimate fat-free mass. Whilst they often lack the sensitivity to differentiate muscle mass from the fat-free mass, they are sometimes used to provide surrogate measures. The reference method for the determination of total-body water is isotopic dilution, in which isotopic tracers are administered and fluid samples taken before and after dosing (see Chapter 2 for further details). The most frequently used isotopes for the determination of total-body water are deuterium and tritium, with deuterium the more common as it is not radioactive. The dilution of ^{14}C-creatine has been proposed as a measure of muscle mass, exploiting the presence of creatine in muscle tissue, as with measuring the urinary excretion of muscle metabolites. However, the ^{14}C-creatine technique does not appear to be in frequent use in man.

Electrical conductance methods such as total-body electrical conductance (TOBEC) and bioelectric impedance analysis (BIA) use the conductive properties of water, and the fact that the water concentration of the fat-free mass is relatively constant at ~72–73 per cent, to provide estimates of the fat-free mass. More advanced BIA models offer estimates of muscle mass using regional measurements and assumed values for the resistivity of muscle mass. However, this approach has yet to be sufficiently validated and, despite its portability and relative ease of use, the method is not in widespread use for the quantification of muscle mass. One reason might be because those who might benefit from such assessment (for instance athletes and the elderly) are also most likely to violate the inherent assumptions of the method, especially with respect to hydration status.

Muscle is a metabolically expensive tissue for the body to maintain. Altering the exercise and nutritional environments enable muscle mass to be gained or sacrificed, in processes which have served our species in its evolutionary past. Today, as we exert greater control on both exercise and nutrition environments, we can confer greater adaptation of muscle. However, optimising muscle mass for functionality is not merely a question of 'more is better' because of the greater energy cost of moving a heavier mass. Under starvation conditions, muscle atrophy reduces the energy requirement. Between these extremes lies an optimal muscle mass for efficient movement and optimal performance. In addition, it is important to highlight the role of the law of specificity – where a muscle recruited will respond to training, while those which are 'dormant' will not. Lastly, although skeletal muscle produces force which facilitates human movement, it cannot do this without the lever system to which it is inextricably linked. This system – the skeleton and its related structures, is the subject of Chapter 6.

References

Cardinale, M., Newton, R. & Nosaka, K. (Eds.) (2011). *Strength and Conditioning: Biological Principles and Practical Applications*. Chichester: Wiley-Blackwell.

Drinkwater, D.T., Martin, A.D., Ross, W.D. & Clarys, J.P. (1986). Validation by cadaver dissection of Matiegka's equations for the anthropometric estimation of anatomical body composition in adult humans. In *Perspectives in Kinanthropometry: The 1984 Olympic Scientific Congress Proceedings, Vol. 1* (edited by J.A.P. Day). Champaign, IL: Human Kinetics, pp. 221–227.

Fleck, S.J. & Kraemer, W.J. (2004). *Designing Resistance Training Programs*. Champaign, IL: Human Kinetics.

Fry, A.C. (2004). The role of resistance exercise intensity on muscle fibre adaptations. *Sports Medicine, 34*, 663–679.

Germann, W.J. & Stanfield, C.L. (2002). *Principles of Human Physiology*. San Francisco, CA: Benjamin Cummings.

Gurney, J.M. & Jelliffe, D.B. (1973). Arm anthropometry in nutritional assessment: nomogram for rapid calculation of muscle circumference and cross-sectional muscle and fat areas. *American Journal of Clinical Nutrition, 26*, 912–915.

Heymsfield, S.B., McManus, C., Smith, J., Stevens, V. & Nixon, D.W. (1982). Anthropometric measurement of muscle mass: revised equations for calculating bone-free arm muscle area. *American Journal of Clinical Nutrition, 36*, 680–690.

Huxley, A.F. & Niedergerke, R. (1954). Structural changes in muscle during contraction: interference microscopy of living muscle fibres. *Nature, 173*, 971–973.

Huxley, H. & Hanson, J. (1954). Changes in the cross-striations of muscle during contraction and stretch and their structural interpretation. *Nature, 173*, 973–976.

Lee, M. & Carroll, T.J. (2007). Cross education: possible mechanisms for the contralateral effects of unilateral resistance training. *Sports Medicine, 37*, 1–14.

Martin, A.D., Spenst, L.F., Drinkwater, D.T. & Clarys, J.P. (1990). Anthropometric estimation of muscle mass in men. *Medicine and Science in Sports and Exercise, 22*, 729–733.

Matiegka, J. (1921). The testing of physical efficiency. *American Journal of Physical Anthropology, 4*, 223–230.

McArdle, W.D., Katch, F.I. & Katch, V.L. (2009). *Exercise Physiology: Nutrition, Energy and Human Performance* (seventh edition). London: Lippincott, Williams & Wilkins.

Pette, D. & Staron, R.S. (2001). Transitions of muscle fiber phenotypic profiles. *Histochemistry and Cell Biology, 115*, 359–372.

Reilly, T. & Waterhouse, J. (2005). *Sport, Exercise and Environmental Physiology*. London: Elsevier.

Wolfe, R.R. (2002). Regulation of muscle protein by amino acids. *The Journal of Nutrition, 132*, S3219–3224.

WHO (World Health Organization). (2007). *Protein and Amino Acid Requirements in Human Nutrition*. Geneva: WHO Technical Report Series 935.

6

BONE TISSUE

Laura Sutton

This chapter will cover:

6.1 Bone anatomy and physiology

The human skeleton is formed by a framework of bones and their associated cartilage. Most adult human skeletons contain 206 bones, which may be classified in a number of ways. The skeletal system serves many important functions, including the provision of shape and support, protection of internal organs, assistance in movement, storage of minerals and blood cell production. In this first section, an overview of the structure and generation of bone tissue is provided. Further detail can be found in any dedicated human anatomy textbook.

6.1.1 Composition and types of bone

Bone is a remarkable material, equalling cast iron in strength, but being one third of the weight and considerably more flexible (Bailey & McCulloch, 1990). It achieves this by combining the high strength and low elasticity calcium hydroxyapatite, with the weaker but more elastic collagen protein, and as a consequence can withstand large forces without breaking. Living bone is predominantly comprised of bone, or osseous, tissue. In addition, it contains other tissue types, including adipose, nervous, epithelial and connective tissues. For this reason, bones are classified as organs. The reference man of the theoretical model

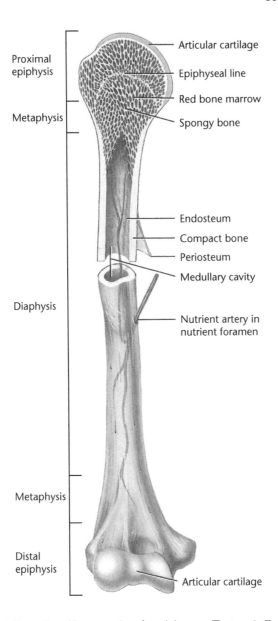

Proximal epiphysis

Articular cartilage

Epiphyseal line

Red bone marrow

Metaphysis

Spongy bone

Endosteum

Compact bone

Periosteum

Medullary cavity

Nutrient artery in nutrient foramen

Diaphysis

Metaphysis

Distal epiphysis

Articular cartilage

FIGURE 6.1 Partially sectioned humerus (arm bone) (source: Tortora & Grabowski (2003). *Principles of Anatomy & Physiology*. Copyright ©2003 by Biological Sciences Textbooks and S.R. Grabowski. Reprinted with permission of John Wiley & Sons, Inc.).

for body composition of Dr Albert Behnke had 14.9 per cent of his body mass made up of bone mass; the corresponding proportion for the reference woman was 12.0 per cent (McArdle, Katch and Katch, 2009).

Individual bones are comprised of cortical (also known as compact or dense) and trabecular (also known as cancellous or spongy) bone tissue, as illustrated in Figure 6.1. Cortical bone tissue is more solid and makes up the hard, outer layer of a bone. The name derives from the Latin *cortex*, meaning the bark of a tree, and is used anatomically to describe the outermost layer of a structure or organ. The bone interior typically comprises trabecular tissue, which is more porous and vascular. The name of the tissue refers to the lattice shape it forms. Given its greater density, cortical bone tissue accounts for a greater proportion of the bone mass within the skeletal system compared to trabecular tissue, but trabecular bone tissue covers a much larger surface area.

The human skeleton may also be divided into its axial and appendicular components. The axial bones include the 80 bones of the skull, vertebral column and thoracic cage. The axial skeleton is so called as it forms the longitudinal axis of the body. The appendicular skeleton consists of the bones comprising the limbs and thoracic and shoulder girdles. The term appendicular has its origins in the word *appendage*, describing the fact that the bones connect to the axial skeleton. The axial skeleton accounts for approximately 40 per cent and the appendicular approximately 60 per cent of the total skeleton.

There are generally considered to be five main types of bone, classified according to their appearance (Table 6.1).

TABLE 6.1 Bone classification according to shape

Type of bone	Description	Example
Short	Short bones tend to be cube-like in appearance and are comprised mainly of trabecular bone	Carpals (wrist)
Long	Mainly comprised of cortical bone tissue, long bones are shaft-like, with articular surfaces at the extremities	Femur (thigh)
Flat	Flat bones are made up of a layer of trabecular bone tissue 'sandwiched' between two layers of cortical bone. They are fairly thin and flat in appearance	Sternum (breastbone)
Irregular	Most bones that do not fit into any of the three preceding categories are labelled irregular bones. They are composed predominantly of trabecular bone tissue	Vertebrae (spine)
Sesamoid	Sometimes classified as short or irregular bones, sesamoid bones are composed of predominantly trabecular bone, and are situated within tendons to increase the mechanical stability and leverage at a joint	Patella (kneecap)

6.1.2 Bone growth and remodelling

Bone tissue is a complex, dynamic tissue that undergoes a life-long process referred to as bone turnover, bone metabolism or bone remodelling. This continuous process involves the removal of mature bone tissue and the generation of new bone tissue. Specifically, the removal of mature bone tissue is termed resorption and is carried out by osteoclast cells, which acidify and proteolytically digest bone. New bone tissue is formed by osteoblast cells, which secrete a substance called osteoid which undergoes mineralisation to form new bone. Osteoblasts that become embedded within the resulting bone matrix are called osteocytes. Together, these osteoclasts and osteoblasts form the 'remodelling units', which systematically replace the entire skeleton, and are illustrated in Figure 6.2.

Throughout infancy and youth, growth hormones stimulate osteoblast activity, resulting in the formation of new bone. Increases in stature occur as a result of increases in the length of long bones. Specifically, cells called chondrocytes form new cartilage at the epiphyseal plates at either end of the bone shaft, elongating the bone. The chondrocytes then perish, allowing osteoblasts to replace them and convert the cartilage to bone tissue. Osteoblasts also lay down new bone tissue on the outer surface, increasing long bone circumference, whilst osteoclasts resorb

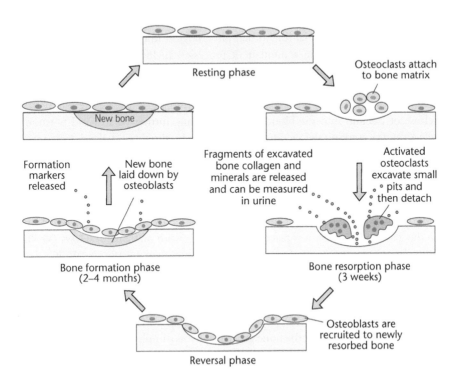

FIGURE 6.2 The bone remodelling cycle (copyright © 1998 *Current Medicine*. Reprinted with permission of SpringerImages).

bone from the inner surface, increasing the diameter of the marrow cavity and reducing the heaviness of the growing bone (Germann and Stanfield, 2002). Eventually, the epiphyseal plates become completely composed of bone tissue, preventing the bones from lengthening further. The bone remodelling cycle still continues throughout adult life, enabling the body to respond to the demands placed upon the skeleton and repair any damage to the bone tissue.

In healthy adults, the processes of bone resorption and formation are closely coupled. The complete basic remodelling cycle takes around three months, with approximately 30 per cent of the skeletal mass renewed each year (Sims and Baron, 2002). Trabecular bone undergoes a more rapid turnover than cortical bone, thus disruptions to the bone remodelling cycle are often more evident at an early stage in the trabecular tissue. A variety of biochemical and mechanical factors regulate the remodelling cycle. Whilst not all of the mechanisms and pathways are completely understood, it has been established that several of the regulatory factors control each other's production, forming feedback loops which influence osteoclast and osteoblast activity, whilst others stimulate local mediators which exert control over skeletal changes (Manolagas, 2000). Two important control loops are hormonal control and mechanical control.

Hormonal control of the remodelling cycle occurs through a negative feedback mechanism, involving parathyroid hormone and calcitonin, which serves to maintain calcium ion homeostasis in the blood (Marieb, 2005). The maintenance of ionic calcium is essential for normal physiological functioning as calcium ions play an important role in a number of processes, including the transmission of nerve impulses and muscle contraction. Parathyroid hormone is released by the parathyroid glands when the level of calcium ions in the blood declines, stimulating osteoclast activity. The process of bone resorption by osteoclasts results in the release of calcium into the bloodstream, inhibiting further parathyroid hormone release and prompting the secretion of calcitonin by the thyroid gland. Calcitonin inhibits the resorption process and prompts bone mineralisation, building bone tissue and reducing the presence of calcium ions in the blood. As blood calcium levels drop, parathyroid hormone release increases again.

Bone remodelling also occurs in response to mechanical stress and gravitational pull. Devised in the late nineteenth century, Wolff's law states that bone will adapt to the load under which it is placed in accordance with mathematical laws (Wolff, 1986 [translation of original German edition published in 1892]). Wolff's law provided an explanation for many observations such as thicker tissue in areas of bone experiencing greater strain, larger bony projections where larger muscles attach to bone, and the bone demineralisation resulting from inactivity. The law has since been refined into the 'mechanostat' model, which is a tissue-level negative feedback system describing the bone growth and loss stimulated by local mechanical elastic bone deformation (Frost, 1987). Elastic deformation refers to the effect of muscle force on bone through voluntary mechanical loading.

Mechanical loading results in the deformation of bone tissue at the site of mechanical stress, stimulating a local adaptive response. The exact mechanism is still uncertain, but it has been suggested that remodelling is directed by electrical signals. Sufficient strain on the bone creates microdamage which stimulates the bone remodelling cycle, as damaged bone tissue must be removed and replaced by healthy tissue. The bone tissue at the site of strain adapts to better cope with the stress placed upon it. Frost (1997) described a 'microdamage threshold range', stating that remodelling can repair damage within the range, but that strains exceeding the range cause too much damage, resulting in bone fracture. Bone modelling works to adjust the bone mass and strength in order that the strain from habitual activities remains below the microdamage threshold. Thus the skeleton optimises the conflicting demands of strength on one hand, and lightness and efficiency of movement on the other.

6.2 Age, gender and lifestyle influences

Although predominantly determined by genetic factors, bone density in adult life is not 'fixed', and may be influenced by hormonal changes, the ageing process, diet and other lifestyle habits. In this section some of the main influential factors are reviewed.

6.2.1 The effects of ageing

The ageing process has adverse effects on the bone compartment. Around middle age, bone resorption begins to exceed formation and a net bone loss occurs with each remodelling cycle. Hormonal changes such as declining levels of oestrogen and testosterone serve to accentuate the imbalance. The sharp decrease in oestrogen associated with the menopause further compounds the situation and women may lose bone mass at an exponential rate following the menopause.

In both men and women, the age-related reductions in muscle mass, strength and functionality result in less mechanical loading of the bones, in turn resulting in reduced bone remodelling. In addition to the ageing process, inactivity contributes to the decline in bone strength. Debilitating postural changes may occur in later life, for example excessive curvature of the thoracic spine, termed 'kyphosis'. Movement becomes more limited and in more severe cases breathing may be impaired and chronic pain experienced.

The most common metabolic disorder affecting the skeletal system is osteoporosis, which is becoming increasingly prevalent as the ageing population expands. Whilst ageing is not the only cause of symptoms of osteoporosis (other causes include, for example, congenital conditions and chronic disuse), it is generally considered an age-related disorder, so is explored here in relation to ageing.

Osteoporosis is characterised by low bone mass and deterioration of the bone tissue, leading to an increased fragility and propensity to fracture. The structural differences between healthy and osteoporotic bone can be observed in Figure 6.3. The term 'osteopoenia' is often used in cases of low bone mass that are not sufficiently severe to be diagnosed as osteoporotic. Descriptions of the diseases and diagnostic criteria are as follows:

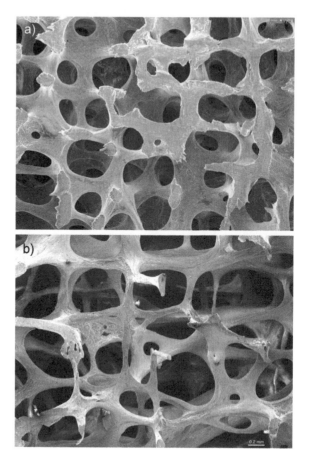

FIGURE 6.3 Comparison of (a) normal and (b) osteoporotic bone architecture (3rd lumbar vertebrae) (copyright © Tim Arnett, University College London).

Osteopoenia – The term 'osteopoenia' may be used to describe low bone mass, but the International Society for Clinical Densitometry (ISCD) lists preferred terms as 'low bone mass' or 'low bone density'. Use of the term 'bone loss' is not recommended unless previous bone mass is known.

Low bone mass is diagnosed when an individual's BMD falls between 1 and 2.5 standard deviations below the corresponding young adult mean value.

In premenopausal women and men under the age of 50, age-adjusted values are preferred (this is especially important for children). Values 2 or more standard deviations below the age-adjusted norm are described as 'below the expected range' (ISCD, 2007).

Osteoporosis – 'a disease characterised by low bone mass and microarchitectural deterioration of bone tissue, leading to enhanced bone fragility and a consequent increase in fracture risk' (Consensus development conference, 1991, as cited in Kanis, Melton, Christiansen, Johnston & Khaltaev, 1994, p.1137).

Osteoporosis is diagnosed when an individual's BMD falls more than 2.5 standard deviations below the corresponding young adult mean value.

Osteoporosis cannot be diagnosed in children, adolescents or men under the age of 50 on the basis of the BMD standard deviation score alone; additional criteria are required, such as low age-adjusted BMD and a clinically significant fracture history (ISCD, 2007).

The risk of falls and incidence of bone fractures has been observed to increase with age. Morbidity and mortality are increased in elderly persons with osteoporotic fractures, particularly those to the hip and spine. The ISCD (2007) now recommends monitoring bone mineral density in women over 65 and men over the age of 70 years irrespective of other risk factors for fracture. Whilst some age-related decline is inevitable, the deleterious effects of ageing on the skeleton can be attenuated by proper nutrition and regular physical activity.

6.2.2 Gender differences

Men and women differ in the relative quantities of many components of body composition, the bone compartment being no exception. Behnke's reference values for young, healthy adults show the average man to have more bone mass than the average woman. The difference extends beyond differences in stature and weight – reference man being the taller and heavier – as when expressed in relative terms, reference man has almost a 3 per cent higher proportion of his overall body mass comprised of bone mass compared to reference woman. Thus, for men and women of similar stature, men will generally have greater bone mass, either due to a larger frame size, greater bone density or both.

Prior to the onset of puberty, boys and girls tend to accrue bone mass at similar rates. The increase in sex hormone secretion during puberty is responsible for the growth spurt that occurs throughout that period. Boys have higher levels of androgens and girls higher levels of oestrogens, both of which stimulate increased osteoblast activity. Much of the differences in size and composition between men and women are accounted for by hormonal differences. Differences in the male and female skeletons begin to emerge, for example the widening of the pelvis in females. The sex hormones are also responsible for the shutdown of growth at the epiphyseal plates, preventing further increases in length. Women generally reach peak bone mass, which may be defined as the maximum quantity of bone tissue at skeletal maturation, earlier than men. Males tend to undergo a longer bone maturation period and usually achieve a greater peak bone mass than women. Peak bone mass is a key determinant of bone mass in later life.

In adulthood, age-related changes in bone mass and density tend to occur at a later stage in men compared to women. It has been well established that women are at a greater risk of osteoporosis than men, and experience a much higher prevalence. The World Health Organization estimated the disease to be three times more common in women than men (WHO, 2003). In conjunction with other factors, the oestrogen deficiency associated with the menopause in women is responsible for a marked reduction in bone mass and density and, in some cases, oestrogen replacement therapy is recommended as a treatment for osteoporosis. Men are still at risk from bone loss and fractures, as age-related decreases in testosterone have a detrimental effect, although the effect is not as pronounced as in women. If fractures do occur, the morbidity in men and women is likely to be similar.

6.2.3 Lifestyle factors

Many lifestyle factors have been purported to exert a deleterious influence on bone health. Whilst the exposition of specific mechanisms is beyond the scope of this chapter, a brief summary of dietary and lifestyle habits commonly associated with effects on the bone compartment is provided.

Alcohol intake

Alcohol consumption is generally regarded as a risk factor for osteoporosis, given frequent findings of low bone mass in alcoholics. Despite this, many studies have reported positive correlations between alcohol intake and bone mass. It may be that at certain levels of consumption, alcohol has negligible or beneficial effects on the skeleton, but that chronic high intakes are detrimental to bone health. Review studies suggest a J-shaped relationship between alcohol consumption and fracture risk (Berg et al., 2008) and U-shaped relationships between alcohol and chronic disease and overall mortality (Klatsky, 2007), implying a slight decrease in risk for moderate drinkers compared to abstainers, but increasing risk at higher levels of alcohol consumption. The exact mechanisms are unknown, but some suggested explanations have been given for research findings.

A possible mechanism by which alcohol may increase bone mass could be through acutely increasing the secretion of calcitonin, a hormone that protects against calcium loss and increases bone mass. Alcohol may also increase levels of oestrogen, which reduces bone resorption. Acute moderate ethanol consumption has been suggested to inhibit bone resorption. Finally, there is a possibility that the phytochemicals present in alcoholic beverages may have a beneficial effect on bone.

Possible explanations for the detrimental effects of high alcohol consumption on bone include the toxic effects of high levels of ethanol, disrupted calcium homeostasis due to an interference with calcium-regulating hormones and decreased osteoblast activity, leading to a reduction in bone formation. Lower BMD may be explained in part by the nutritional deficiencies often present in heavy drinkers. In addition, the greater risk of fracture reported in alcoholics may be partly attributable to an increased frequency of falls.

Carbonated and/or caffeinated beverages

It has been suggested that bone mineral density is inversely correlated with the consumption of carbonated and/or caffeinated beverages; however, much of the evidence is equivocal. The phosphate and other sweeteners present in some soda drinks have been suggested to impede calcium absorption, but conclusive evidence is lacking. Caffeine has a slight depressant effect on calcium absorption and has been purported to reduce bone mass and increase the risk of fracture. However, it is likely that the deleterious effect of caffeine on the bone compartment has been overstated.

Heaney (2002) reported that the negative effect of caffeine on calcium absorption is sufficiently small to be offset fully by just one to two tablespoons of milk, and that there was no substantial effect of caffeine on total 24-hour calcium excretion. Following a review of the literature, Heaney concluded that there is no evidence that caffeine has any harmful effect on bone status or on the calcium economy in individuals who ingest the current recommended daily intake of calcium.

The Framingham Osteoporosis Study (Tucker et al., 2006) and the Oslo Health Study (Høstmark, Søgaard, Alvær and Meyer, 2011) both found inverse associations between the consumption of cola drinks and bone mineral density, but found conflicting results regarding the intake of non-cola soft drinks. Some authors have concluded that it is the fact that carbonated beverages may displace healthier beverages, particularly those containing calcium, that leads to an association with lower BMD, rather than any direct effects of the drinks themselves.

Micronutrient intake

Calcium is one of the primary constituents of bone mineral and approximately 99 per cent of the calcium stores in the human body are found within bone tissue. However, the body cannot store excess calcium as it can fat, for example, and calcium is regularly excreted. Therefore, a frequent dietary intake is required. The levels of calcium consumed are generally shown to be positively correlated with bone mass, but there remains some contention in the literature. Evidence of a direct relationship between dietary calcium intake and bone mass is not always apparent; it may be that there is a particular level of intake beyond which the beneficial effects of calcium are attenuated. However, it is widely accepted that inadequate dietary calcium impairs bone development in early life, and it has been suggested that a low calcium intake throughout childhood and adolescence increases the risk of osteoporosis in adulthood.

Studies in which calcium supplements are given often report increases in bone mass, particularly when baseline calcium intake is low. Research demonstrates that increased intakes often reduce bone loss, with most studies conducted on vulnerable groups such as postmenopausal women. Given the pivotal role of calcium in maintaining bone health, the adverse effects of low calcium consumption during early life and its potential to reduce age- and menopause-related bone loss in later life, a high dietary intake of calcium is likely to be beneficial at all ages.

In addition to calcium, a constant supply of phosphate salts is essential to normal bone growth and maintenance. Other minerals such as fluoride, iron, magnesium and zinc are also required. An adequate vitamin intake is important, particularly vitamins A, B_{12}, C, D and K, all of which play a role in bone formation and the maintenance of a healthy bone structure.

Protein intake

Dietary protein intake plays a role in the maintenance of bone health, and both cross-sectional and intervention studies have shown positive associations between dietary protein intake and bone density. High protein intakes increase serum insulin-like growth factor 1 – also known as mechano growth factor – levels, promoting osteoblast activity (Dawson-Hughes, 2003). The role of protein in the building and maintenance of muscle mass may also play a role, as muscle and total body mass are positively related to bone density. High protein diets have also been shown to attenuate total and trabecular bone loss during periods of weight loss. Some concerns have been voiced over high protein diets, as a high protein intake is associated with increased urinary calcium excretion; however, a high protein intake also increases calcium absorption, which may serve to protect bone tissue.

Smoking

Smoking has an adverse effect on bone mineral density and has been shown to be associated with greater fracture risk, poorer healing post-fracture and increased risk of osteoporosis (Sloan, Hussain, Maqsood, Eremin and El-Sheemy, 2010). Smoking as a risk factor appears to be independent of age and weight, and the development of low bone mass and osteoporosis may be accelerated in both men and women. Passive smoking has also been associated with low bone mass.

The detrimental effects of cigarette smoking are generally dose-dependent. Chemicals from tobacco smoke cause cellular damage, and blood vessel constriction reduces the delivery of oxygen and nutrients to the bone tissue. In addition, smokers may be less physically active, drink more alcohol and have poorer diets than non-smokers, increasing the risks of damage to the bone compartment. Women who smoke tend to produce less oestrogen and may experience early menopause, further increasing the risk of low bone mass.

The detrimental effects of smoking on bone health may, at least partially, be reversible. Smoking-related bone loss may be reduced by cessation, particularly in conjunction with the modification of other lifestyle risk factors.

6.3 Response to physical activity and exercise

Changes in bone mass, architecture (the structure and orientation of bone) and strength occur in response to impact loading and exercise. Such responses are referred to as functional adaptations, and occur in response to mechanical loading, in particular compressive impact forces, but also tensile forces exerted on the tendon attachment sites as muscles contract, and inertial forces imposed by total and segmental mass under the influence of gravity. Responses to mechanical activity improve the ability of the body to cope with the demands of the activity and give greater protection against injury. The beneficial influences of physical activity on bone are evident across the age spectrum, as bone mass and strength increase in young adulthood, whilst age-related bone loss may be minimised in the elderly.

Both cross-sectional and longitudinal studies have shown the responses to physical activity and exercise to be site-specific, meaning that adaptive changes will occur at the sites of mechanical stress. Thus, the responses to different activities differ. The more vigorous the activity, the more pronounced the functional adaptation will be. In the present section, responses to different sporting and occupational activities are described, and the effects of decreasing loading on the bone or overtraining are examined.

6.3.1 Effects of different sporting activities

Due to the site-specific nature of bone formation and the dose-dependent response to mechanical stress, different sporting activities effect different changes in the skeleton. The largest responses will be seen in high-impact activities and those which require exposure to heavy loading, for example Olympic weightlifting, which places large loads on the skeleton. Bone density increases and the tendon attachment sites increase in size and strength. The site-specific responses to strain are particularly noticeable in sports in which one limb is dominant. For example, bone mineral content and density have been shown to be substantially greater in the dominant arm compared to the non-dominant arm in tennis players and athletes of throwing events.

Endurance athletes such as long-distance runners undergo repeated loading, but their lighter body weight, smaller musculature and lower absolute strength means they require less bone mass and strength compared to strength and power athletes, so the skeletal response is less pronounced. The microdamage associated with the repeated impact from predominantly lower-body activities such as running can stimulate remodelling in the lower body, but responses are generally not evident in the upper body. Overall bone mass and density may be increased in endurance athletes compared to non-athletes, provided the athletes are not in negative energy balance.

Activities that do not involve high impact loading may not effect large changes in bone mass and density. Whilst there may be some effect on bone tissue of repetitive muscular action, the frequency of the pull against the bone tissue appears to be less important than the magnitude for stimulating adaptation. For example, swimming and cycling are not high-impact loading activities, and the lack of weight-bearing results in lower skeletal responses than those seen in activities in which greater loads are placed on the skeleton. In a comparison of elite male runners, cyclists, triathletes and controls, Stewart & Hannan (2000) found that cycling was associated with low bone mineral density (the mean T-score at the lumbar spine was -1.16, which falls in the osteopoenic range), whereas running was associated with greater bone mineral density. In athletes who performed both, the influence of running appeared prevalent.

In addition to the differences in the bone compartment observed between distinct sports, differences also exist between similar sports, for example between different football codes or different playing positions within a particular team sport, due to slightly different loading patterns. For example, rugby forwards tend to demonstrate greater bone mass than backs due to greater impact loading and the tendency for players in forward positions to have greater lean and total body mass (Elloumi et al., 2009).

Weight cycling occurs when athletes cannot maintain their 'competition weight' year round, but allow their weight to fluctuate during the season, achieving their desired weight during important competitions and allowing their weight to increase during 'off-season' periods. Weight cycling, in particular rapid weight loss, has been shown to exert a negative effect on bone mass and athletes in weight-controlled sports or sports in which weight and appearance play an important role may be at risk of poor bone health due to weight cycling or restricted energy intakes. Examples of such sports include those in which participants are classified by weight, for example combative sports; aesthetic sports, such as dancing and gymnastics; and sports in which body weight is kept low in order to benefit performance, for example horse racing. The effects of dietary restrictions on bone are addressed in more detail in Section 6.3.4, with a particular focus on female athletes.

6.3.2 Physically demanding occupations

Responses to mechanical loading occur not just in response to exercise, but also habitual activity as occurs in physically demanding occupations. Tasks that cause mechanical loading of the skeleton include lifting, locomotion or climbing whilst supporting external loads and other activities in which the body is lifted repeatedly against gravity. Bone strength is important for coping with physical strain and also for the prevention of injury that may contribute to poor performance and time away from the workplace. Examples of occupations in which bone strength is advantageous and may be increased as a result of work-related activity include manual labour, such as construction work, and active roles in the military.

Military training, as with other forms of repetitive exercise, results in increased bone formation in both men and women. However, fracture risk is an important consideration, as prolonged marches and novel exercise may result in stress fractures. Armstrong, Rue, Wilckens & Frassica (2004) reported that approximately 5 per cent of military recruits experience stress fracture injuries during infantry training. The authors suggested possible contributing factors to be the regular, intense physical training combined with substantial, acute weight loss. Stress fractures are known to occur more frequently in female cadets than male cadets, which may be partly due to women generally having smaller, less dense bones. Finestone and Milgrom (2008) reported that enforcing a minimum sleep regimen and reducing the amount of cumulative marching during training substantially decreases the risk and severity of stress fractures, without adversely affecting performance.

6.3.3 Effects of overtraining

The stress fractures mentioned in the previous section provide a common example of overuse injury. Such fractures are defined as partial or complete fractures resulting from repetitive loading, and occur more frequently with excessive training frequency and insufficient recovery time. The bone remodelling cycle is unable to repair the microdamage at the rate at which it occurs and bone mass is unable to increase in response to the mechanical strain. If microdamage accumulates at a particular site of loading, the area becomes weak and susceptible to fracture. The shin and ankle are common sites of stress fracture. Another common complaint is medial tibial stress syndrome, colloquially known as 'shin splints', where tenderness and pain are felt on the medial tibia. Tibial stress syndrome may progress to a stress fracture if the repetitive loading continues.

Hormonal responses to overtraining include elevated production of the stress hormone cortisol and lower production of the sex hormones, signalling a reduction in the formation of new bone which, if prolonged, leads to decreased bone mass and density and a higher risk of fracture. The features of the female athlete triad described in the next subsection also provide an example of symptoms of the overtraining syndrome.

6.3.4 The female athlete triad

The term female athlete triad is used to describe a combination of three interrelated conditions sometimes observed in female athletes or females participating in high amounts of recreational exercise: disordered eating, amenorrhoea and osteoporosis, as illustrated in Figure 6.4. Each one of the three conditions can be associated with serious health consequences, and the appearance of all three increases the risk of morbidity and rate of mortality. Girls and women exhibiting one condition of the triad should be screened for the remaining conditions.

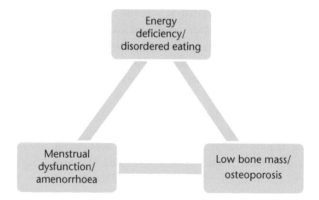

FIGURE 6.4 The female athlete triad.

Disordered eating can range from mild caloric restriction to potentially fatal eating disorders, such as anorexia nervosa. Given the tendency for sportswomen to exhibit relatively low levels of body fat compared to the general population, eating disorders may go undetected. The term 'anorexia athletica' has been proposed to describe female athletes who demonstrate disturbances in eating behaviour, but may not necessarily meet all the criteria for clinical diagnosis of an eating disorder.

Amenorrhoea is defined as the absence of menstrual periods. Primary amenorrhoea is the failure to establish menstruation by the expected time of menarche (the first menstrual period), whereas secondary amenorrhoea occurs when menstrual cycles cease post-menarche. Menstrual dysfunction is known to occur more frequently in female athletes than in the general female population. Generally, at least three months without menstruation are required for a diagnosis of secondary amenorrhoea.

The third condition forming the triad is osteopoenia/osteoporosis, as defined previously. When bone density falls lower than the age-related expectation, the risk of stress fractures and musculoskeletal injury is increased. The mechanical stress of regular physical activity further increases the likelihood of bone fracture or other injuries. Low bone mass and density during early adulthood can be detrimental to bone health in later life, and the likelihood of early osteoporosis post-menopause is increased.

The three disorders are interrelated and the presence of one may trigger or exacerbate another. For example, the reduction in body mass associated with disordered eating reduces the magnitude of the loading forces acting on the skeleton during everyday life, and dietary deficiencies and hormonal disruptions have an adverse effect on the bone remodelling cycle. Total body mass and its constituent lean and fat masses are related to bone density, and low body mass is recognised as a risk factor for osteoporosis. In female athletes with low body fat, the maintenance or increase of lean mass could help protect against low bone mass and osteoporosis. Bone mineral density is often lower in amenorrhoeic athletes compared to those with normal menstrual function, even in the absence of differences in body composition, suggesting that oestrogen levels play an important role in the osteoporosis component of the female athlete triad. Whilst the relationship between low body fat and amenorrhoea is well established, causality has yet to be established definitively.

All three disorders need not be present for a woman's health to be compromised; furthermore, problems may occur without the full conditions being developed, for example, restricted dietary intake may result in a low energy availability without disordered eating habits being identified, hormonal irregularities may exist without amenorrhea, or bone density may be reduced without the diagnostic criteria for osteoporosis being met. Female athletes particularly vulnerable to the triad include those competing in aesthetic events such as ballet, endurance events such as long-distance running, and other events in which a thin body shape or low body weight are viewed as advantageous.

6.3.5 *Effects of inactivity*

Degenerative changes in the skeleton occur as a result of deloading and inactivity. The functional adaptations to long-term physical training are no longer required when training is ceased. Excess bone tissue undergoes resorption, causing gradual declines in density and strength toward pre-training levels. The lack of loading brought about by periods of inactivity such as injury, bed-rest or microgravity also result in imbalances in the bone remodelling cycle which cause bone mass and density to decrease. According to Tan (2006), in the clinical setting, bone density is reduced by approximately 40–45 per cent following 12 weeks of bed-rest, and by the thirtieth week, over 50 per cent bone density may be lost. Such bone loss is termed 'disuse osteoporosis', and is accelerated in patients with neurogenic paralysis. In recognition of the likelihood of fracture amongst elderly individuals, programmes of osteogenic exercises have been established and have proven effective in retarding the bone loss, or even adding bone (Kerr, Ackland, Masalen, Morton & Prince, 2001).

In microgravity environments such as the environment experienced during space flight, the weight supported by the bones is negligible and movement does not effect the same mechanical loading. As a result, processes similar to those associated with bed-rest can occur, and may do so at a faster rate. Those undertaking prolonged space flight must perform specific exercises in order to prevent disuse osteoporosis. Most lost bone mass should be regained upon return to earth, although if significant bone deterioration has occurred, astronauts must be cautious when exercising, as their fracture risk will be greater, and the time required to recover from injury may be longer.

6.4 Estimation of bone density *in vivo*

Whilst often used interchangeably, the terms 'bone density' and 'bone mineral density' are not synonymous. Bone density refers to a volumetric, i.e. three-dimensional, density ($g.cm^{-3}$), whereas bone mineral density is in fact an areal, i.e.

two-dimensional, quantity (g.cm^{-2}). In this section, current methods for the assessment of bone mass and density are reviewed.

6.4.1 Dual X-ray absorptiometry (DXA)

Dual X-ray absorptiometry was developed as a method of bone densitometry, which is defined as a quantitative measurement of bone mass or density. It is sometimes referred to as quantitative digital radiography (QDR). As outlined in Chapter 2, the differential attenuation of two X-ray beams is used to provide a measure of areal bone mineral density and projected bone area, from which the bone mineral content can be estimated. Today, DXA provides the criterion method for bone densitometry and is used in the clinical assessment of bone mineral status, in particular the diagnosis of conditions associated with low bone mineral content/ density such as osteoporosis. Diagnostic scans are usually conducted on specific sites associated with high mortality risk following fracture, such as the proximal femur and lumbar spine, or the forearm if the hip/spine region is inaccessible.

Bone mineral density values are compared to a large reference database incorporated into the DXA software, producing T- and Z-scores. The T-score is the deviation from a gender-matched standard for peak bone mineral density, and the Z-score provides a score based on reference data taking into account gender and age. The standard deviation scores allow for the identification of low bone mass and osteoporosis (diagnostic criteria are provided in Section 6.2.1).

In addition to diagnostic scans, DXA can provide bone mineral density values for the body as a whole or other defined regions of interest. T-scores and Z-scores can be produced for the whole body, but do not serve as a diagnostic tool in adults, rather a general indicator of bone mineral status. Peripheral DXA may be used to make rapid, peripheral measurements at sites such as the finger or the heel. In addition to the quantitative assessment of bone mineral content and density, DXA may be used to make qualitative assessments, for example lateral spine scans produce images of the vertebrae that enable the visual assessment of vertebral compression or fracture.

6.4.2 Quantitative computed tomography (QCT)

Quantitative computed tomography (QCT) is a densitometric method capable of providing volumetric measurements of bone density. The method also enables the segmentation of bone tissue into its constituent cortical and trabecular tissues. The ability to isolate trabecular bone tissue is advantageous, as the high turnover in trabecular bone results in a faster response to disease or intervention. Therefore, the method is highly sensitive to changes in the bone compartment.

The QCT method may be used in the evaluation of osteoporosis, with most assessments made at the lumbar spine. However, QCT incurs a greater radiation exposure and is more costly than DXA, so is less frequently used in screening and monitoring. Scans tend to be reserved for cases in which DXA scans are difficult to interpret and a higher sensitivity and accuracy are warranted. Example of such cases include the assessment of bone (mineral) density in individuals with osteoarthritis or a spinal deformity such as scoliosis. In addition to QCT assessments, standard CT scanners may be used to provide whole-body scans. Peripheral QCT may be used for peripheral measurements such as forearm scans.

6.4.3 Quantitative ultrasound (QUS)

An alternative approach to radiographic techniques is provided by quantitative ultrasound (QUS). The absorption of a high-frequency sound wave is used to assess fracture risk, as ultrasound velocity is related to trabecular bone density. Assessment by QUS is typically made at the heel, or sometimes the shin, as it is not possible to measure higher risk sites such as the femur and lumbar spine. Standard ultrasonography may also be used to provide data on bone 'quality'. Ultrasound bone densitometry does not involve radiation exposure and may be useful as a cost-effective screening method, but is unlikely to replace radiographic methods as a 'gold standard' densitometric approach.

6.4.4 Alternative methods

Assessments of bone mineral density could be made by the predecessor to DXA, dual-photon absorptiometry (DPA). The DPA method involves the measurement of the attenuation of photon beams produced by a radionuclide source, whereas DXA uses a stable X-ray tube. The radioactive source in DPA instruments decays, requiring replacement, without which accuracy and precision decrease. Thus, the cost of maintenance is higher and the results less clinically useful.

Standard radiographs (X-rays) may be used to image bone tissue and are often used for fracture assessment. However, conventional X-ray techniques are not as sensitive to changes in the bone mineral compartment as DXA and CT, and a large amount of bone mass must be lost in order for changes in bone density to be detected. Furthermore, effective X-ray doses from standard radiographs are higher than those produced by DXA.

Single X-ray absorptiometry (SXA) may also be used to measure bone mineral density. Assessments are typically made at peripheral sites such as the wrist or heel. During SXA scans, the region undergoing assessment must be immersed in a water bath in order to simulate uniform tissue thickness. The SXA method is less frequently used than DXA and is generally considered an inferior technique.

Magnetic resonance imaging (MRI) can be used to image bone tissue and assess density and fracture risk. It provides a useful alternative to CT and DXA for individuals who are unable to undergo exposure to ionising radiation, for example pregnant women. Other advantages to MRI include the ability to estimate volumetric bone density, and the fact that high resolution images allow the assessment of trabecular bone structure. However, MRI scans are more costly and take longer to acquire and, whilst soft-tissue images are generally more detailed than CT images, MRI images of bony structures tend to be less detailed.

Conclusion

In conclusion, whilst predominantly determined by genetic factors, bone tissue is labile and can adapt in response to behavioural habits. In parallel with optimising the level of fatness and muscular strength, lifelong impact loading exercise is likely to optimise bone density. As we have seen, the issues relating to diminished bone density are not the sole prevail of the elderly, but affect athletes in several sports where intensive training undermines the mechanisms by which the body maintains its health. Whilst some decline in bone health is inevitable with advancing age, the adverse effects of the ageing process can be attenuated through the maintenance of a healthy lifestyle from a young age.

References

Armstrong III, D.W., Rue, J.H., Wilckens, J.H. and Frassica, F.J. (2004). Stress fracture injury in young military men and women. *Bone, 35*, 806–816.

Bailey, A.D. & McCulloch, R.G. (1990). Bone tissue and physical activity. *Canadian Journal of Sport Sciences, 15*, 229–239.

Berg, K.M., Kunins, H.V., Jackson, J.L., Nahvi, S., Chaudry, A., Harris, K.A. et al. (2008). Association between alcohol consumption and both osteoporotic fracture and bone density. *The American Journal of Medicine, 121*, 406–418.

Dawson-Hughes, B. (2003). Calcium and protein in bone health. *The Proceedings of the Nutrition Society, 62*, 505–509.

Elloumi, M., Ounis, O.B., Courteix, D., Makni, E., Sellami, S., Tabka, Z. et al. (2009) Long-term rugby practice enhances bone mass and metabolism in relation with physical fitness and playing position. *Journal of Bone and Mineral Metabolism, 27*, 713–720.

Finestone, A. and Milgrom, C. (2008). How stress fracture incidence was lowered in the Israeli army: a 25-yr struggle. *Medicine and Science in Sports and Exercise, 40*, S623–S629.

Frost, H.M. (1987). The mechanostat: a proposed pathogenic mechanism of osteoporoses and the bone mass effects of mechanical and nonmechanical agents. *Bone and Mineral, 2*, 73–85.

Frost, H.M. (1997). Why do marathon runners have less bone than weight lifters? A vital biomechanical view and explanation. *Bone, 20*, 183–189.

Germann, W.J. and Stanfield, C.L. (2002). *Principles of Human Physiology*. San Francisco, CA: Benjamin Cummings.

Heaney, R.P. (2002). Effects of caffeine on bone and the calcium economy. *Food and Chemical toxicology, 40*, 1263–1270.

Høstmark, A.T., Søgaard, A.J., Alvær, K. and Meyer, H.E. (2011). The Oslo Health Study: a dietary index estimating frequent intake of soft drinks and rare intake of fruit and vegetables is negatively associated with bone mineral density. *Journal of Osteoporosis* [ePublication ahead of print].

ISCD (International Society for Clinical Densitometry). (2007). *ISCD Official Positions*. West Hartford, CT: ISCD.

Kanis, J.A., Melton III, L.J., Christiansen, C., Johnston, C.C. and Khaltaev, N. (1994). The diagnosis of osteoporosis. *Journal of Bone and Mineral Research, 9*, 1137–1141.

Kerr, D., Ackland, T., Masalen, B., Morton, A. & Prince, R. (2001). Resistance training over 2 years increases bone mass in calcium replete postmenopausal women. *Journal of Bone and Mineral Research*, 16, 175–181.

Klatsky, A.L. (2007). Alcohol, cardiovascular diseases and diabetes mellitus. *Pharmacological Research, 55*, 237–247.

Manolagas, S.C. (2000). Birth and death of bone cells: basic regulatory mechanisms and implications for the pathogenesis and treatment of osteoporosis. *Endocrine Reviews, 21*, 115–137.

Marieb, E.N. (2005). *Anatomy & Physiology* (second edition). San Francisco, CA: Pearson.

McArdle, W.D., Katch, F.I. and Katch, V.L. (2009). *Exercise Physiology: Nutrition, Energy and Human Performance* (seventh edition). London: Lippincott, Williams & Wilkins.

Sims, N. and Baron, R. (2002). Bone: Structure, function, growth and remodeling. In R.H. Fitzgerald, H. Kaufer, and A. L. Malkani (Eds.) *Orthopaedics* (pp. 147–159). St. Louis, MI: Mosby Inc.

Sloan, A., Hussain, I., Maqsood, M., Eremin, O. and El-Sheemy, M. (2010). The effects of smoking on fracture healing. *The Surgeon, 8*, 111–116.

Stewart, A.D. & Hannan, J. (2000). Bone density in cyclists, runners and controls. *Medicine and Science in Sports and Exercise, 32*, 1373–1377.

Tan, J.C. (2006). *Practical Manual of Physical Medicine and Rehabilitation* (second edition). St Louis, MI: Elsevier Mosby.

Tucker, K.L., Morita, K., Qiao, N., Hannan, M.T., Cupples, L.A. and Kiel, D.P. (2006). Colas, but not other carbonated beverages, are associated with low bone mineral density in older women: The Framingham Osteoporosis Study. *American Journal of Clinical Nutrition, 84*, 936–942.

Wolff, J. (1986). *The Law of Bone Remodeling*. Berlin: Springer [translation of original German edition, 1892].

WHO (World Health Organization). (2003). *Prevention and Management of Osteoporosis*. Geneva: WHO Technical Report Series 921.

7

ANTHROPOMETRIC SURROGATES FOR FATNESS AND HEALTH

Mike Marfell-Jones, Alan M. Nevill and Arthur D. Stewart

This chapter will cover:

7.1   Indices of stature and mass
7.2   Girths, girth indices and other measurements
7.3   Skinfolds
7.4   Best practice approach to measuring
7.5   ISAK protocols for skinfolds and selected other measures
7.6   Statistical methods for identifying the optimal body shape for health and physical performance

In Chapter 3, portable methods for estimating fatness were discussed, which included the prediction of fatness from equations, validated against a laboratory method. In this chapter, we will concentrate on the use of raw data, or derivatives of it, to produce surrogate values for fatness, without recourse to calculating fat mass or percentage fat.

7.1 Indices of stature and mass

Throughout biological systems, there is a need to quantify body size in order to interrelate an array of influences affecting an organism. In humans, body mass, defined as the quantity of matter in the body (measured by weight, i.e. mass multiplied by the force of gravity) and stature (measured by standing height) are the most frequently used size variables. Each can be used individually, or in a basic algorithm relating the two. In adults, mass is much more variable than stature, and therefore more influential in a variety of indices that combine both measures. Other dimensional measurements, for example leg length, frame size or muscularity, can be included to consider other aspects of the phenotype as discussed in Chapter 4. This chapter, however, will focus on adiposity.

Mass change is used as an outcome variable in a range of clinical and nutritional applications. However, the degree to which it represents, or misrepresents, adiposity has been the subject of protracted debate. In dietary interventions, the composition of mass lost (which invariably includes fat-free tissue, especially glycogen and water, in addition to fat) is contingent on initial composition, diet and the rate of weight loss (Hall, 2007). In addition, we have to consider the nature and receptiveness of any individual to different exercise stimuli that have consequences for body composition which are mode- and age-dependent. Exercise can slow the rate of muscle loss, or trigger muscle mass gain, as discussed in Chapter 5. However, simply focusing on total body mass could obscure commensurate muscle gain and fat loss, which in some circumstances cancel one another out. As a consequence, it is important to consider a range of indices beyond mass which are more informative.

The virtue of any ratio of measures reflecting adiposity is related to its correlation with fatness as measured by a reference method. The strength of this correlation is, therefore, contingent upon not only the range of values in the index measured, but also the robustness of the criterion method and the nature of the sample assessed. In this respect, much of the material in the public domain can be misleading, because it fails to satisfy one or more of these criteria. Indices of stature and mass are themselves affected by the magnitude and variability of each component (as discussed in Section 7.6).

The ratio of mass to stature is commonly referred to as the weight-height ratio, and is simply mass divided by stature. (Note that there is scope for confusion between this and waist-height ratio which is more common.) Alternatively, the stature can be divided by the cube root of mass to give what is commonly known as the *ponderal index*. (The reciprocal of this is used in the ectomorphy calculation for somatotype (as described in Chapter 4).) The popularity of both these indices declined largely due to the acceptance of the alternative ratio of mass (in kilograms) divided by the square of stature (in metres). This third ratio, proposed by Belgian astronomer and mathematician Adolphe Quetelet (1796–1874) and initially known as the Quetelet Index, endures today as the Body Mass Index (or BMI). The theoretical rationale for a taller person being heavier is sound, but rests heavily on the premise that the BMI maximally correlates with mass, and minimally correlates with stature (Billewicz, Kemsley & Thomson, 1962).

The BMI readily attracted widespread acceptance because reference ranges were developed and applied globally. However, it also received criticism on a number of counts. First, like the other ratios which only use stature and mass, it presumes that excessive weight is attributable solely to adiposity, with the consequence that individuals who are large-framed, well-muscled or have proportionately long torso and short legs, can be misrepresented as fatter than they actually are. The World Health Organization and most public health authorities use BMI as surrogate for fatness, with the resulting misclassification of many individuals whose body structures are far from the norm. For example, it is well recognised that ethnicity exerts a strong influence on relative proportions, frame size and musculature, and these elements are reflected in differential relationships of fatness with BMI (Rush et al., 2007). As a consequence, it has been necessary to introduce ethnic-specific cut-offs in order to use the BMI in different populations (WHO, 2004). Equally, the issues of men and women using the same cut-off values and the rating of growing children have triggered much controversy. For example, in a study of nearly 19,000 adults, BMI related better to surrogates for muscularity than to frame size or skinfolds (Ross et al., 1988). Converting the observed correlation between BMI and skinfold total into the *predictive index* $PI = 100 \times [1-((1-r^2)^{0.5})]$, the authors calculated a figure of just 21.5 per cent (only 15.8 per cent better than pure chance), leading them to conclude that the BMI's utility in assessing fatness was 'more misleading than informative' (p. 172). Despite the BMI's higher correlation with skinfold-corrected girth, it still proved insufficient to make individual predictions of muscle mass with any confidence.

Attempts to adjust the BMI to produce a more relevant index at an individual level have included the Fat-Free Mass Index (FFMI) (Kouri, Pope, Katz & Oliva, 1995). This involves using measured percentage fat in a regression model and deriving an index which has been used to assess muscularity, both in muscle wasting and the likelihood of achieving certain levels of musculature by pharmacological intervention. This is an interesting approach, but relies on the selection of measures to assess percentage fat which are invariably less accurate than commonly appreciated. Issues related to muscle mass are discussed in more detail in Chapter 5.

7.2 Girths, girth indices and other measurements.

Waist girth is perhaps the most widely recognised simple measure as generally reflective of adiposity and is logically used for this purpose because it is well-established that abdominal obesity exerts an additive and independent influence on health risk. However, measurements in overweight individuals are notoriously difficult to acquire, and different protocols for waist measurement produce disparate results which are greater in females (Wang et al., 2003), and across the 'waist zone' (from the iliac crest to the tenth rib), appear much more variable than previously thought (Stewart, Nevill, Stephen & Young, 2010). Aside from this, waist girth does not discriminate between subcutaneous and the more-harmful visceral fat. It had been previously suggested that waist circumference and BMI independently contributed to abdominal fatness, and that the combination of BMI and waist girth explain more of the variation in non-abdominal, abdominal subcutaneous and visceral fat than BMI alone (Janssen, Heymsfield, Allison, Kotler & Ross, 2002). Subsequently, it was suggested that, within BMI categories, increasing waist girth was associated with greater health risk, and that waist girth (uncorrected) outperformed BMI in predicting health risk when considered separately (Janssen, Katzmarzyk & Ross, 2004). This latter study considered BMI and waist girth data from nearly 15,000 adults from the NHANES III survey by calculating odds ratios for the obesity-related health disorders of hypertension, dyslipidemia and factors other than high waist girth defining the metabolic syndrome (plasma lipid, glucose, blood pressure). After adjusting for confounding variables, the authors demonstrated that, at any waist girth level, individuals had broadly similar health risk, irrespective of their BMI status.

Hip girth has also been used as an individual measurement predictor and, like waist girth, is problematic to measure in overweight or obese individuals. Because of the focus of health-risk research on abdominal obesity favouring measurements of waist girth or the waist:hip ratio, consideration of hip girth alone has been relatively neglected, despite the hip being a key storage site for excess adipose tissue, especially in women. In a study of 75 postmenopausal women aged 45–76 years, hip girth explained 74 per cent of the variance in total fat and 85 per cent of the variance in abdominal fat, as assessed by dual X-ray absorptiometry (DXA) (Raja, Hansen, Baber & Allen, 2004). The authors were attempting to predict abdominal adiposity and related their findings to the BMI cut-off value of $25\,kg.m^{-2}$. This study added some useful information to current knowledge for this particular population, and concluded that the cut-off points for the healthy:overweight dichotomy corresponded to a hip girth of 100 cm, and a fat:fat-free tissue ratio within the pelvic abdominal region of 1.0, as defined by DXA analysis. A much larger cohort study of 1,462 women aged 38–60 was undertaken in 1968 and followed up for total mortality, myocardial infarction, cardiovascular disease and diabetes 24 years later in 1992 by Lissner, Bjorkelund, Heitmann, Seidell & Bengtsson (2001). Their findings showed hip circumference to be significantly and independently associated with risk, but that larger hip girths were, to some extent, protective of health – in line with previous findings that narrow hips (after adjusting for waist size) were associated with greater diabetes risk (Seidell, Han, Feskens & Lean, 1997). The mechanism for this association is not clear, but may relate to hips being an alternative site for excess fat disposal as an alternative to the abdominal region, for which the association with health risk is well established. The apparent contradiction in findings between these studies needs, however, to be interpreted with caution. It might not be appropriate to compare pre- and post-menopausal women using a similar analogy, because of the centralisation of body fat distribution which is known to occur after the menopause.

Arm girth has been used historically as a substitute for body weight in protein-calorie malnutrition, using a single girth measure in childhood (Vijayarghavan & Gowrinath Sastry, 1976). Unfortunately, this fails to quantify tissue masses as it assumes that muscle wasting will be associated with minimal body fatness. The measurement of arm girth alone in other groups, such as athletes or the elderly, requires an adjustment for skinfold thickness. Using a concentric circular model, subtraction of the skinfold multiplied by π from the arm girth generates a theoretical muscle girth readable with a nomogram (Gurney & Jelliffe, 1973). The same approach has been used to adjust leg girth (Jones & Pearson, 1969), thigh girth (Tothill & Stewart, 2002) and calf girth (Stewart, Stewart & Reid, 2002). The issue of how to adjust for overlying adipose tissue is important for estimates of motor function or fat-free tissue, even though uncorrected thigh girth has been used, like hip girth, to assess ischemic heart disease risk (Kahn, Austin, Williamson & Arensberg, 1996) and premature death (Heitmann & Frederiksen, 2009). An increased thigh circumference, if uncorrected, could reflect either an increase in thigh muscle or an increase in femoral fat accumulation, which could reflect increasing or decreasing functional capacity, respectively.

The waist-to-hip ratio (WHR) is the most commonly-used girth ratio, and its value reflects clear differences between gynoid and android profiles (which are described in Chapter 1). A study of 30,000 adults from 52 countries across all continents investigated risk of myocardial infarction and concluded that nine risk factors collectively accounted for 90 per cent of the attributable risk in men and 94 per cent in women (Yusuf et al., 2004). Subsequent consideration of the anthropometric data, which confirmed that the waist-to-hip ratio was the obesity measure with the strongest association consistently across different groups, led to the suggestion that use of BMI as the measure of obesity was obsolete as it underestimated the health consequences of obesity (Kragelund & Omland, 2005). Waist-to-stature ratio (WSR) has also been shown to be a helpful index in an epidemiological study from Hong Kong (Ho, Lam & Janus, 2003). This study considered BMI, waist circumference (WC), WHR and WSR in relation to cardiovascular risk factors in 2,895 Chinese adults. Using receiver operator characteristic analysis of 21 risk factors, the WSR showed the greatest predictive potential for most factors in both men (13 of 21) and women (10 of 21) with cut-off values of 0.48 applying to both. This led the researchers to recommend the straightforward message – that 'one's waist circumference should not exceed half one's stature' (p. 683). However, some caution may be warranted in applying this unilaterally. As identified in Chapter 4, males and females do not necessarily have the same BMI/shape relationships, and ethnic variation in shape within a BMI category profoundly alters health risk (WHO, 2004), between individuals of similar size. A similar proposition might be applied to hip girth, which, arguably, is more influenced by skeletal breadth than waist girth.

Attempts to combine measures of abdominal adiposity with mass and stature resulted in the Conicity Index (CI) $CI = Waist\ Girth\ /\ [0.109 \times (mass\ /\ stature)^{0.5}]$, with both waist girth and stature expressed in metres (Valdez, 1991). Modelling the body as a shape between that of a cylinder and a double cone, whereby fatter individuals have a larger CI and a more 'biconal' shape due to abdominal fat accumulation, is theoretically sound. However, the CI has experienced only modest use in epidemiological research. It was found to be the method of choice for coronary risk screening in a Brazilian study of 968 adults (Pitanga & Lessa, 2005), but performed less well than BMI as a marker for predicting coronary heart disease incidence and mortality in over 4,000 individuals screened longitudinally as part of the Framingham Heart Study (Kim, Owen, Williams & Adams-Campbell, 2000). In addition, the CI performed less well than waist girth in predicting abdominal adiposity in children (Taylor, Jones, Williams & Goulding, 2000).

The sagittal abdominal diameter (SAD) is a further example of an anthropometric measurement gaining acceptance in a range of studies for assessing abdominal obesity. Referred to variously as abdominal height, abdominal thickness or anterior-posterior abdominal depth, the measure is the linear distance across the abdomen in the mid-sagittal plane. An early investigation demonstrated its utility (and that of its ratio to the coronal diameter) in assessing visceral fat changes in men (van der Kooy, Leenen, Seidell, Deurenberg & Visser, 1993). A large cohort study of a multi-ethnic population established the SAD as a consistent predictor of coronary heart disease risk across all ages, sexes and racial groups, even though it was more strongly associated with this risk in the younger age group of 18–44 years (Iribarren, Darbinian, Lo, Fireman & Go, 2006). A study of 83 middle-aged adults of mixed ethnicity (type II diabetics and healthy controls) assessed SAD in the supine position and showed that it, together with age, best predicted an adverse metabolic profile, (Valsamakis et al., 2004), the authors considering anterior-posterior-axis fat deposition to be more hazardous to health than lateral fat deposition. The rationale for using the SAD is that it appears to be more sensitive to visceral fat accumulation. A pilot study of shape change in relation to weight loss, demonstrated that SAD change explained 91 per cent of weight loss in obese men – more than for any other anthropometric variable, including waist girth (Stewart, Nevill & Johnstone, 2009). The validity of a circular model to estimate visceral fat had previously been called into question in an MRI study of 35 individuals with a wide range in abdominal adiposity (He et al., 2004). An elliptical model using internal sagittal and coronal diameters was found to be superior to a circular model in predicting visceral fat area, both in terms of explained variance and prediction residuals. However, some caution is necessary in interpreting results which sample the abdomen in a single slice. A study of anti-retroviral drugs in treating human immunodeficiency virus used CT scans of the abdomen at nine locations spanning L2–3, L3–4 and L4–5 (Ellis et al., 2007), in 24 adults from three distinct ethnicities. The results showed a difference in visceral to subcutaneous adipose tissue ratio (VAT/SAT) by site. At L2–3, referring to the second and third lumbar vertebrae, the mean ratio was 1.8, but reduced to 0.9 at L4–5. Significant intra- and inter-site differences were seen from the L3–4 region moving in an inferior direction. The use of single slices (which are frequently used in body composition research in order to reduce cost or radiation exposure) may therefore constitute undersampling of the complex distribution of visceral fat, and potential consequences for misinterpretation – which goes some way to explaining the conflicting findings which prevail in the literature.

Assembling what is known from medical or public health studies and the most commonly used surrogates for adipose tissue, several clear messages become apparent. There is no universally accepted measure or ratio for predicting adiposity or health, despite the fact that various studies perpetuate the use of BMI, waist girth and WHR. As well as the profound male-female differences in VAT/SAT, there are also clear ethnic differences. For example, Asian Indians have been observed to have smaller waists, but greater visceral fat than European Caucasians of similar BMI (Raji, Seely, Arky & Simonson, 2001), which explains why diabetes risk in Asians rises rapidly within the normal healthy ranges of waist or BMI for Europeans. It is also clear that, anatomically, fat distribution can vary markedly over even a short distance, highlighting the importance of attention to detail in measurement protocols and reliability.

7.3 Skinfolds

Skinfolds differ from the dimensional measures above, in that they specifically assess adipose tissue. Skinfolds are linear measurements of a double fold of compressed adipose tissue plus associated skin depth. As a measure of total adiposity, skinfolds have been used in large numbers of prediction equations over the years, with percentage fat as the dependent variable. Researchers should be wary, however, of such predictions, given that, for intersubject comparisons, their accuracy relies on the validity of five assumptions in making the translation from the linear distance across a skinfold to percentage fat. For an equation to have validity, skinfolds need to be of constant compressibility; skin thickness needs to be the same at all sites, the fat fraction of adipose tissue needs to be constant; adipose tissue patterning needs to be constant; and the ratio of external to internal adiposity needs to be constant. None of these assumptions hold true as has been demonstrated by Clarys, Martin, Drinkwater & Marfell-Jones (1987), among others.

The ratio of external to internal adiposity, for example, is an important consideration because, with increasing adiposity, there is commonly an increase in the proportion of fat situated internally. Accepting that the body does not have a uniformly thick layer of superficial adipose tissue, the depth at representative sites can, nevertheless, provide an indication of regional 'fat topography' or patterning. While skinfolds have traditionally been considered to derive percentage fat, their use as raw data can equally, if not better, be used in other ways to assess adiposity. These include recording individual skinfolds, the total of a series of skinfolds, the ratio of two skinfolds or groups of skinfolds, and computing the average skinfold depth across a number of sites. This approach avoids most of the assumption errors associated with converting skinfolds into percentage fat, and is being used increasingly in assessing athletes, in whom the assumptions of constant density and proportions of the constituents of the fat-free mass are most tenuous. Skinfolds alone, however, measuring, as they do, subcutaneous adipose tissue, take no consideration of visceral fat, which becomes more abundant in fatter individuals and, as highlighted previously, constitutes the greater health risk.

The use of multiple skinfolds offers an effective way to describe fat patterning. One way of conveying such information is to plot a skinfold map – a radial plot of the sites measured. Figure 7.1 illustrates two examples of very lean athletes measured using the eight ISAK-recommended sites.

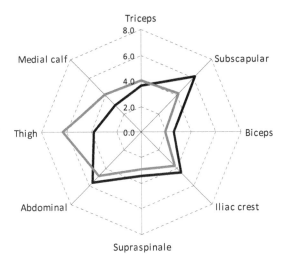

FIGURE 7.1 Skinfold map depicting extreme leanness in male (dark) and female (light) endurance athletes.

Alternatively, skinfolds can be used to calculate ratios, which can be graphed (examples of which are illustrated in Figure 7.2), to describe the centralisation of adipose tissue associated with growth, ageing, and abdominal obesity. For example, research which monitored five trunk and five extremity skinfolds during childhood and adolescence demonstrated a profound shift in their ratio (i.e. trunk:extremity), with sexual dimorphism most marked after age 12 years (Malina & Bouchard, 1988).

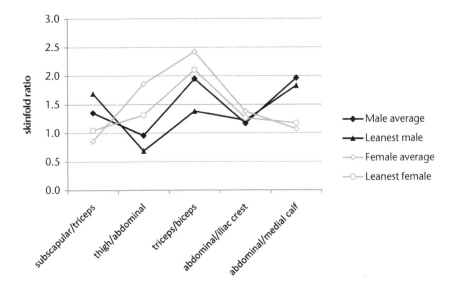

FIGURE 7.2 Skinfold ratios, depicting the progress towards extreme leanness.

7.4 Best practice approach to measuring

As mentioned in Chapter 1, a 1–2 per cent diurnal variation in stature is observed as a function of spinal loading according to the orientation of the spine (Tyrell, Reilly & Troup, 1985). This loading reduces stature after the person rises, and is reversed when retiring to bed. Combining this with the alteration in body mass as a function of eating, drinking, urinating, defecating, breathing and perspiring and a different pattern ensues. The mass increases throughout the day while the stature decreases, and this alters the 'true' BMI, as indicated in Figure 7.3.

Diurnal variation in BMI is largely ignored in public health literature, despite the fact that this variation is commonly around 1 kg.m^{-2} in an adult, and exceeds this in children. This is a particular concern for children whose BMI, when plotted on the trajectory chart, may be subject to change by as much as 35 centiles as a consequence. In reality, most children are likely to be measured during school hours, but, still, the measurement time of day has a strong influence and should be recorded on the pro forma sheet.

Considerable skill is required to measure skinfolds proficiently, and this is best acquired through structured training and practice. By permission, the 2011 ISAK protocol has been reproduced (in part) in Section 7.5 to illustrate the approach that has greatest international acceptance of any single set of anthropometric measures. The standards adopted by ISAK include tightly defined protocols, structured training and exam-based certification which quantifies intra-, and, more importantly, inter-measurer technical error of measurement. All too often in the literature, individual laboratories either fail to report error statistics entirely or quantify only intra-measurer error.

While views differ on protocols, approaches and even which side of the body is measured, the requirement for landmarking is fundamental to minimising location errors. Despite this, many early studies did not undertake landmarking, and

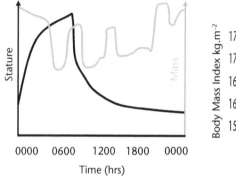
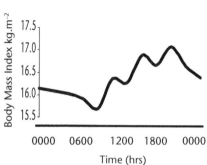

FIGURE 7.3 Left: Schematic diagram of fluctuations in stature (dark) and mass (light) over 24 hours. Right: Actual change in BMI from measured stature and mass in a five-year-old child (Stewart, unpublished data).

interpretation of their data quality should be judged accordingly. In previous decades, measuring skinfolds without landmarking was the common practice, and because it was recognised that there was considerable error associated with the technique, it was argued that fine location of skinfolds constituted 'mistaken exactitude' (Durnin, 1997, p. 1042). However, more recently, evidence to the contrary has confirmed that, even in highly experienced measurers, as little as 1 cm deviation in the measurement site can produce significantly different results (Hume & Marfell-Jones, 2008). However, of the eight ISAK sites these authors compared, some varied less than others, none were free of differences between a central measuring point and eight peripheral points 1 cm away, and one, the abdominal site, was different at all eight peripheral points.

Care must also be exercised with the sequence in which measurements are taken, in order to avoid measurer-influenced error arising from knowledge of the measurement value obtained on the previous immediate measuring occasion. Such error can be reduced by the use of a recorder and the measuring of the day's full battery of measures twice right through in sequence before taking any necessary third measures.

7.5 ISAK protocols for skinfolds and selected other measures

Here, we provide ISAK protocols for stretch stature, all eight skinfold sites, four girths and anterior-posterior abdominal depth (sagittal abdominal diameter). This is a reduced measurement set from the ISAK full profile (updated in 2011; and omitting flexed arm girth and bone breadths from the restricted profile) which has been assembled for the purpose of adipose tissue prediction with the permission of ISAK. Some landmark detail has been incorporated in order for the definitions to be more easily understood.

Stretch stature

Definition: The perpendicular distance between the transverse planes of the Vertex and the inferior aspect of the feet.
Subject position: The subject stands with the heels together and the heels, buttocks and upper part of the back touching the scale. The head, when placed in the Frankfort plane, need not be touching the scale. The Frankfort plane is achieved when the Orbitale (the lower edge of the eye socket) is in the same horizontal plane as the Tragion (the notch superior to the tragus of the ear). When aligned, the Vertex is the highest point on the skull.
Method: Having positioned the head in the Frankfort plane, the measurer relocates the thumbs posteriorly towards the subject's ears, and far enough along the line of the jaw of the subject to ensure that upward pressure, when applied, is transferred through the mastoid processes. The subject is then instructed to take and hold a deep breath and while keeping the subject's head in the Frankfort plane the measurer applies gentle upward lift through the mastoid processes. The recorder

assists by watching that the heels do not leave the floor and that the position of the head is maintained in the Frankfort plane. The recorder then places the head board firmly down on the Vertex, compressing the hair as much as possible. The measurement is taken before the subject exhales.

Triceps skinfold (see Figure 7.4A)

Definition: The skinfold measurement taken parallel to the long axis of the arm at the point on the posterior surface of the arm, in the mid-line, at the level of the marked mid-acromiale-radiale landmark.

Subject position: The subject assumes a relaxed standing position with the right arm hanging by the side and the hand in the mid-prone position.

Method: Palpation of this site (where the mid-line of the posterior surface of the arm meets the projected mid-acromiale-radiale perpendicular to the arm's long axis) is recommended before measurement.

Subscapular skinfold (see Figure 7.4B)

Definition: The skinfold measurement taken with the fold running obliquely downwards at a point 2 cm along a line running laterally and obliquely downward from the undermost tip of the inferior angle of the scapula.

Subject position: The subject assumes a relaxed standing position with the arms hanging by the sides.

Method: The line of the skinfold is determined by the natural fold lines of the skin, and is commonly at about a 45° angle.

Biceps skinfold (see Figure 7.4C)

Definition: The skinfold measurement taken parallel to the long axis of the arm at the point on the anterior surface of the arm at the level of the mid-acromiale-radiale landmark, in the middle of the muscle belly.

Subject position: The subject assumes a relaxed standing position with the right arm hanging by the side and the hand in the mid-prone position.

Method: Palpation of this site (where a vertical line in the middle of the muscle belly when viewed from the front meets the projected mid-acromiale-radiale) is recommended before measurement.

Iliac crest skinfold (see Figure 7.4D)

Definition: The skinfold measurement taken immediately above the most superior point on the iliac crest where a line drawn from the mid-axilla (middle of the armpit), on the longitudinal axis of the body, meets the ilium.

Subject position: The subject assumes a relaxed standing position. The right arm should be either abducted or placed across the trunk.

Method: The line of the skinfold generally runs slightly downward posterior-anterior, as determined by the natural fold lines of the skin.

Supraspinale skinfold (see Figure 7.4E)

Definition: The skinfold measurement taken at the intersection of the line from the marked Iliospinale to the anterior axillary border and a horizontal line at the level of the marked Iliocristale.

Subject position: The subject assumes a relaxed standing position with the arms hanging by the sides.

Method: The fold runs medially downward and anteriorly at about a 45° angle as determined by the natural fold of the skin.

Abdominal skinfold (see Figure 7.4F)

Definition: The skinfold measurement taken vertically at the point 5 cm horizontally to the right-hand side of the omphalion (midpoint of the navel).

Subject position: The subject assumes a relaxed standing position with the arms hanging by the sides.

Method: It is particularly important at this site that the measurer is sure the initial grasp is firm and broad, since often the underlying musculature is poorly developed. This may result in an underestimation of the thickness of the subcutaneous layer of tissue. *Note*: Do not place the fingers or caliper jaw inside the navel.

Front thigh skinfold (see Figure 7.4G)

Definition: The skinfold measurement taken parallel to the long axis of the thigh at the Front Thigh skinfold site (mid way between the Patellare and the Inguinal Point).

Subject position: The subject assumes a seated position at the front edge of the box with the torso erect, the arms supporting the hamstrings and the leg extended.

Method A: The measurer stands facing the right side of the subject on the lateral side of the thigh. The skinfold is raised at the marked site, and the measurement taken.

Method B: Subjects with particularly tight skinfolds are asked to assist by lifting the underside of the thigh, and if this proves insufficient, the recorder (standing on the subject's left) assists by raising the fold, with both hands, at about 6 cm either side of the landmark. The measurer then raises the skinfold at the marked site and takes the measurement.

Medial calf skinfold (see Figure 7.4H)

Definition: The skinfold measurement taken vertically at the point on the most medial aspect of the calf at the level of the maximal girth.

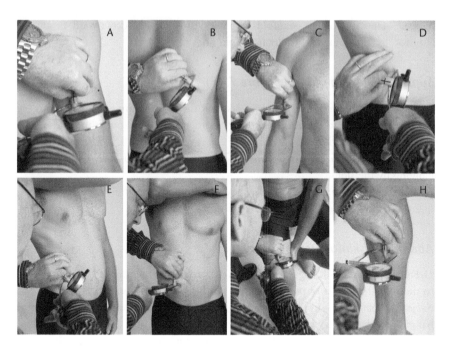

FIGURE 7.4 ISAK skinfold measurements. (A) triceps; (B) subscapular; (C) biceps; (D) iliac crest; (E) supraspinale; (F) abdominal; (G) thigh; and (H) medial calf.

Subject position: The subject assumes a relaxed standing position with the right foot placed on the box. The right knee is bent at about 90°.

Method: With the subject's right foot on the box and the calf relaxed, the fold is raised parallel to the long axis of the leg. *Note*: Remember the landmark is located and marked with the body weight equally distributed on both legs, but the skinfold measurement is made with the right knee flexed to 90° in order to reduce muscle tension, making the fold easier to measure.

Arm girth

Definition: The circumference of the arm at the level of the mid-acromiale-radiale site, perpendicular to the long axis of the arm.

Subject position: The subject assumes a relaxed standing position with the arms hanging by the sides. The subject's right arm is abducted slightly to allow the tape to be passed around the arm.

Method: Once the cross-taped position has been achieved, the tape should be aligned so that the mid-acromiale-radiale landmark is situated centrally between the two parts of the tape.

Waist girth

Definition: The circumference of the abdomen at its narrowest point between the lower costal (tenth rib) border and the top of the iliac crest, perpendicular to the long axis of the trunk.

Subject position: The subject assumes a relaxed standing position with the arms folded across the thorax.

Method: The anthropometrist stands in front, or at the side, of the subject, who abducts the arms slightly, allowing the tape to be passed around the abdomen. The stub of the tape and the housing are then both held in the right hand while the anthropometrist uses the left hand to adjust the level of the tape at the back to the adjudged level of the narrowest point. The anthropometrist resumes control of the stub with the left hand and, using the cross-handed technique, positions the tape in front at the target level. With the subject breathing normally, the measurement is taken at the end of a normal expiration (end tidal). If there is no obvious narrowing of the waist, the measurement is taken at the mid-point between the lower costal (tenth rib) border and the iliac crest.

Hip girth

Definition: The circumference of the buttocks at the level of their greatest posterior protuberance, perpendicular to the long axis of the trunk.

Subject position: The subject assumes a relaxed standing position with the arms folded across the thorax. The subject's feet should be together and the gluteal muscles relaxed.

Method: The anthropometrist passes the tape around the hips from the side. The stub of the tape and the housing are then both held in the right hand while the anthropometrist uses the left hand to adjust the tape to the adjudged level of the greatest posterior protuberance of the buttocks. The anthropometrist resumes control of the stub with the left hand, and, using the cross-hand technique, positions the tape at the side, checking that it is held in a horizontal plane at the target level, before taking the measurement.

Calf girth

Definition: The circumference of the leg at the level of the medial calf skinfold site, perpendicular to its long axis.

Subject position: The subject assumes a relaxed standing position with the arms hanging by the sides. The subject's feet should be separated with the weight evenly distributed. (The subject usually stands in an elevated position, e.g. on an anthropometric box, to make it easier for the measurer to align the eyes with the tape.)

Method: The anthropometrist passes the tape around the calf and then slides the tape to the correct plane. The stub of the tape and the housing are both held in the right hand while the anthropometrist uses the left hand to adjust the level of the tape to the marked level. The anthropometrist resumes control of the stub with the left hand and, using the cross-hand technique, positions the tape so that it is held in a plane perpendicular to the axis of the leg. The tape is then readjusted as necessary to ensure it has not slipped and does not indent the skin.

Anterior-posterior abdominal depth (sagittal abdominal diameter)

Definition: The horizontal linear distance in the sagittal plane between the point on the skin surface of the abdomen immediately inferior to the omphalion with maximal anterior extension and the corresponding dorsal surface of the torso.

Subject position: The subject assumes a relaxed standing position with the arms folded across the chest and continues breathing normally.

Method: The measurer stands to the side of the subject and extends the side branches of the large sliding calipers holding the calipers so that the measurer's thumb is on top of the caliper blade and not between the blades as this may restrict the ease of measurement. (Note that extensions on the caliper blades are not used for this measurement and may need to be removed entirely.) Maintaining the calipers horizontally, place the edge of one caliper blade on the anterior skin surface immediately inferior to the omphalion at the most anterior protuberance, and slowly close the other blade until it meets the skin surface superficial to the lumbar spine, as depicted on the front cover of this book. (With some subjects the caliper blade will contact the skin superficial to the dorsal musculature, leaving a concavity.) Follow the normal breathing pattern of the subject for at least two full cycles, and record the measurement at end-tidal expiration, ensuring the caliper blades are not indenting the skin surface. Subjects are encouraged to relax completely and not to contract the abdominal muscles (thereby artificially reducing the measurement. (*Note:* If the omphalion is below the level of the fifth lumbar vertebra, the measurement is taken horizontally from the level of the base of the fifth lumbar spinous process to a corresponding point on the anterior surface of the abdomen).

7.6 Statistical methods for identifying the optimal body shape for health and physical performance

Human physique consists of three distinct, but interrelated, anthropometric components: (1) body size, (2) body composition and (3) structure or shape (Slaughter & Christ, 1995). Body size refers to the physical magnitude of the body and its segments (stature, mass, surface area etc.). Body composition consists of the amount of various constituents in the body such as fat, muscle, bone etc. Body structure, or shape, describes the distribution of body parts expressed as ratios, such as the body mass index (BMI), the inverse ponderal index or the head length-to-body length (exclusive of head) ratio. The latter concept of shape was discussed by Mosimann (1970), who defined the term 'shape' as the ratio of two body dimensions measured in the same units in order to yield a 'dimensionless' ratio. The crural index (simplistically defined as the leg length below the knee divided by the leg length above the knee) is a typical example. The purpose of this section, therefore, is to outline a number of statistical methods that can be used to predict the optimal human body shape for a variety of health and physical performance functions.

Optimal shape predictor of health measures

Human body shape is a valuable source of information about health, nutritional status and the risk of disease. At present, only a few indices of shape are used in clinical practice and epidemiology, both of which still rely primarily on the BMI. Despite the widespread criticism it has received, there is compelling evidence to suggest that increased risk of mortality is associated with either high or extremely low BMI (Durazo-Arvizu, McGee, Li & Cooper, 1997).

But why is BMI (Mass / Height^2) and not some other mass-by-height ratio, for example the Ponderal Index (Mass / Height^3), better associated with mortality? Based on the principle of geometric similarity, the Ponderal Index should be theoretically independent of body size. If both high and low body fat is the likely cause of increased mortality, we need to adjust body mass to reflect fat or adiposity, independent of body size. This could be achieved by scaling body mass to be independent of height.

Based on the original model proposed by Quetelet (1869), $M = a.H^2$, Benn (1971) proposed the following simple generalisation, $M = a.H^p$, to render body mass (M) independent of height (H), where p is chosen to best suit the population under study. The model can be linearised with a log-transformation and a regression analysis on $\log_e(M)$, using $\log_e(H)$ as a predictor, to estimate the unknown parameter (p). Nevill & Holder (1995) calculated the height exponents (p) when fitting the model to n = 2,366 Allied Dunbar national fitness survey (ADNFS) subjects by age group vs. gender. These are illustrated in Table 7.1.

TABLE 7.1 The height exponents (p) scaling weight for differences in height by age and gender (n= 2366)

Age group (y)	16–24	25–34	35–44	45–54	55–64
Male	2.52	1.71	1.66	1.72	2.08
Female	1.93	1.89	1.66	1.46	1.42

Clearly, p is considerably less than 3, much closer to the value 2 (median 1.72) adopted by the index BMI.

Confirming that adiposity should scale to BMI, Nevill, Stewart, Olds and Holder (2006) explored the relationship between skinfold caliper readings (S) and body size (using body mass, M, and stature, H), at eight sites and between four sports plus controls, using the following proportional allometric model

$$S = a \cdot H^{b_1} \cdot M^{b_2} \cdot \exp(c.age + d.age^2) \qquad (7.1)$$

The model can be linearised with a log-transformation that will naturally overcome the positive skewness in such data. (Note that empirically-derived stature, H^{b_1}, and mass terms, M^{b_2}, can be expressed as $M^{b_2} H^{b_1} = (M / H^{-b_1/b_2})^{b_2}$, a ratio not dissimilar to the body mass index $BMI = M / (H^2)$ provided b_1 / b_2 is approximately -2.) This model appeared reasonable at the majority of sites for both male and female subjects, suggesting that a power function of BMI^{b_2} is the optimal body-size index associated with skinfold measurements.

The same proportional allometric model (with allometric body size components) was proposed and fitted to the ADNFS systolic and diastolic blood-pressure results (Nevill et al., 1997). After a logarithmic transformation, the parsimonious solution was able to confirm that b_1 / b_2 was close to -2 for both systolic and diastolic blood pressure, once again identifying the optimal predictor of blood pressure as BMI.

In summary, the optimal body-mass-to-height ratio associated with various health measures appears to be $BMI = mass / height^2$ (kg / m^2). However, with the recent development of three-dimensional scanners, as mentioned in Chapters 2 and 4, a wider range of body girth measurements and their ratios will become available to the research community that may, in future, identify more effective shape indicators of health risk and mortality.

Optimal shape predictor of physical performance

There are limited studies investigating the association between body shape and physical performance. One such article by Tanaka & Matsuura (1982) identified the Ponderal index as a key predictor of 10,000 m running performances of 114 Japanese young, middle- and long-distance runners (age $= 19.0 \pm 1.7$ years). Similar findings were reported by Nevill, Tsiotra, Tsimeas & Koutedakis (2009a) when investigating most appropriate body-shape characteristics associated with a variety of physical performance measures (e.g. 20 m shuttle, 40 m sprint and vertical jump test) in Greek children. The authors adopted the same proportional allometric model used in equation (7.1) above. The results suggest that the reciprocal Ponderal index (RPI) ($RPI = height / mass^{0.333}$), rather than BMI, is the most appropriate body-shape indicator associated with running and jumping activities.

Further support for the reciprocal Ponderal index comes from a study by Nevill, Holder & Watts (2009b) which investigated the body size, shape and age characteristics of successful professional footballers. The results identified that, despite a significant increase in professional footballers' height, body mass and BMI from 1973–1974 to 2003–2004, no differences in the body shape parameter, RPI or age were identified. However, when players from successful teams (top six) were compared with less-successful teams using binary logistic regression, players from successful teams were found to be taller and more linear, as identified by a greater RPI and Ectomorphy score (both $P<0.05$) and also younger ($P<0.05$) – a trend that appears to have increased in the most recent season studied, 2003–2004, and a characteristic that also appears greater amongst forwards ($P<0.05$).

In conclusion, the optimal human body-shape index associated with, and used to detect health risk appears to be BMI = (mass / height^2). In contrast, the optimal body-shape index associated with physical performance involving running, jumping and multiple sprint sports, such as soccer, appears to be the reciprocal Ponderal index RPI = (height / mass$^{0.333}$). With any index that seeks to summarise the body's complexity, errors are inevitable, and great caution is warranted in interpreting data for individuals. However, for larger samples and populations, such indices are convenient, and useful, provided their limitations are appreciated. Despite a wider range of potentially new indices coming from 3D scanners in the future, at present BMI and RPI appear to continue to provide a valuable indication of optimal shape associated with health and physical performance respectively.

References

Benn, R.T. (1971). Some mathematical properties of weight-for-height indices used as measures of adiposity. *British Journal of Preventive and Social Medicine, 25*, 42–50.

Billewicz, W.Z., Kemsley, W.F.F. & Thomson, A.M. (1962). Indices of adiposity. *British Journal of Preventive & Social Medicine, 16*, 183–188.

Clarys, J.P., Martin, A.D., Drinkwater, D.T. and Marfell-Jones, M.J. (1987). The skinfold: myth and reality. *Journal of Sports Sciences, 5*, 3–33.

Durazo-Arvizu, R., McGee, D., Li, Z. & Cooper, R. (1997). Establishing the nadir of the body-mass index mortality relationship: a case study. *Journal of the American Statistical Association, 92*, 1312–1319.

Durnin, J.V.G.A. (1997). Skinfold thickness measurement (reply). *British Journal of Nutrition, 78*, 1042–1043.

Ellis, K.J., Grund, B., Visnegarwala, F., Thackeray, L., Miller, C.G., Chesson, C.E. et al. for the strategies for management of anti-retroviral therapy (SMART) study group. (2007). *Obesity, 15*, 1441–1447.

Gurney, J.M. & Jelliffe, D.B. (1973). Arm anthropometry in nutritional assessment: nomogram for rapid calculation of muscle circumference and cross-sectional muscle and fat areas. *American Journal of Clinical Nutrition, 26*, 912–915.

Hall, K.D. (2007). Body fat and fat-free mass inter-relationships: Forbes's theory revisited. *British Journal of Nutrition, 97*, 1059–1063.

He, Q., Engelson, E.S., Wang, J., Kenya, S., Ionescu, G., Heymsfield, S.B. & Kotler, D.P. (2004). Validation of an elliptical anthropometric model to estimate visceral compartment area. *Obesity Research, 12*, 250–257.

Heitmann, B.L. & Frederiksen, P. (2009). Thigh circumference and risk of heart disease and premature death: prospective cohort study. *British Medical Journal, 339*, ePub b3292 doi:10.1136/bmj.b3292

Ho, S-Y., Lam, T-H. & Janus, E.D. for the Hong Kong Cardiovascular Risk Factor Prevalence Study Steering Committee (2003). Waist to stature ratio is more strongly associated with cardiovascular risk factors than other simple anthropometric indices. *Annals of Epidemiology, 13*, 683–691.

Hume P. & Marfell-Jones, M. (2008). The importance of accurate site location for skinfold measurement. *Journal of Sports Sciences, 26*, 1333–1340.

Iribarren, C., Darbinian, J.A., Lo, J.C., Fireman, B.H. & Go, A.S. (2006). Value of the sagittal abdominal diameter in coronary heart disease risk assessment: cohort study in a large, multiethnic population. *American Journal of Epidemiology, 164*, 1150–1159.

Janssen, I., Heymsfield, S.B., Allison, D.B., Kotler, D.P. & Ross, R. (2002). Body mass index and waist circumference independently contribute to the prediction of nonabdominal, abdominal subcutaneous and visceral fat. *American Journal of Clinical Nutrition, 75*, 683–688.

Janssen, I., Katzmarzyk, P.T. & Ross, R. (2004). Waist circumference and not body mass index explains obesity-related health risk. *American Journal of Clinical Nutrition, 79*, 379–384.

Jones, P.R. & Pearson, J. (1969). Anthropometric determination of leg fat and muscle plus bone volumes in young male and female adults. *Journal of Physiology, 204*, 63P–66P.

Kahn, H.S., Austin, H., Williamson, D.F. & Arensberg, D. (1996). Simple anthropometric indices associated with ischemic heart disease. *Journal of Clinical Epidemiology, 49*, 1017–1024.

Kim, K.S., Owen, W.L., Williams, D. & Adams-Campbell, L.L. (2000). A comparison between BMI and conicity index on predicting coronary heart disease: The Framingham Heart Study. *Annals of Epidemiology, 10*, 424–431.

Kouri, E.M., Pope Jr., H.G., Katz, D.L. & Oliva, P. (1995). Fat-free mass index in users and nonusers of anabolic-androgenic steroids. *Clinical Journal of Sports Medicine, 5*, 223–228.

Kragelund, C. & Omland, T. (2005). A farewell to body-mass index? *The Lancet, 366*, 1589–1591.

Lissner, L., Bjorkelund, C., Heitmann, B.L., Seidell, J.A. & Bengtsson, C. (2001). Larger hip circumference independently predicts health and longevity in a Swedish female cohort. *Obesity Research, 9*, 644–646.

Malina, R.M. & Bouchard, C. (1988). Subcutaneous fat distribution during growth. In C. Bouchard & F.E. Johnston (Eds.) *Fat Distribution During Growth and Later Health Outcomes* (pp. 63–84). New York: Alan R. Liss.

Mosimann, J.E. (1970). Size allometry – Size and shape variables with characterizations of lognormal and generalized gamma distributions. *Journal of the American Statistical Association, 65*, 930–945.

Nevill, A.M. & Holder, R.L. (1995). Body mass index: a measure of fatness or leanness? *British Journal of Nutrition, 73*, 507–516.

Nevill A.M., Holder R.L., Fentem, P.H., Rayson, M., Marshal,l T., Cooke, C.B. et al. (1997). Modelling the associations of BMI, physical activity and diet with arterial blood pressure: some results from the Allied Dunbar national fitness survey. *Annals of Human Biology, 24*, 229–247.

Nevill, A.M., Holder, R.L. & Watts, A.S. (2009b). The changing shape of 'successful' professional footballers. *Journal of Sports Sciences, 27*, 419–426.

Nevill A.M., Stewart, A.D., Olds, T. & Holder, R.L. (2006). The relationship between adiposity and body size reveals the limitations of BMI. *American Journal of Physical Anthropology, 129*, 151–156.

Nevill, A.M,, Tsiotra, G., Tsimeas, P. & Koutedakis, Y. (2009a). Allometric associations between body-size, shape and physical performance of Greek children. *Paediatric Exercise Science, 21*, 220–232.

Pitanga, F.J.G. and Lessa, I. (2005). Anthropometric indexes of obesity as an instrument of screening for high coronary risk in adults in the city of Salvador-Bahia. *Arquivos Brasileros de Cardiologia, 85*, 26–31.

Quetelet, L.A. (1869). *Physique Sociale, Vol. 2* (p. 92). Brussels: C. Muquardt.

Raja, C., Hansen, R., Baber, R. & Allen, B. (2004). Hip girth as a predictor of abdominal obesity in post menopausal women. *Nutrition, 20*, 772–777.

Raji, A., Seely, E.W., Arky, R.A. & Simonson, D.C. (2001). Body fat distribution and insulin resistance in healthy Asian Indians and Caucasians. *Journal of Clinical Endocrinology and Metabolism, 86*, 5366–5371.

Ross, W.D., Crawford, S.M., Kerr, D.A., Ward, R., Bailey, D.A. & Mirwald, R.M. (1988). Relationship of the body mass index with skinfolds, girths and bone breadths in Canadian men and women aged 20–70 years. *American Journal of Physical Anthropology, 77*, 169–173.

Rush, E.C., Goedecke, J.H., Jennings, C., Micklesfield, L., Dugas, L., Lambert, E.V. et al. (2007). BMI, fat and muscle differences in urban women of five ethnicities from two countries. *International Journal of Obesity, 31*, 1232–1239.

Seidell, J.C., Han, T.S., Feskens, E.J.M. & Lean, M.E.J. (1997). Narrow hips and broad waist circumferences independently contribute to increased risk of non-insulin-dependent diabetes mellitus. *Journal of Internal Medicine, 242*, 401–406.

Slaughter, M.H. & Christ, C.B. (1995). The role of body physique assessment in sport science. In N.G. Norgan (Ed.). *Body Composition Techniques in Health and Disease.* Cambridge: Cambridge University Press.

Stewart, A.D., Nevill, A.M. & Johnstone, A.M. (2009). Shape change assessed by 3D laser scanning following weight loss in obese men. In P.A. Hume & A.D. Stewart (Eds.) *Kinanthropometry XI: 2008 Pre-Olympic Congress Anthropometry Research* (pp. 20–24). Auckland: Sport Performance Research Institute New Zealand, Auckland University of Technology.

Stewart, A.D. Nevill, A.M., Stephen R. & Young, J. (2010). Waist size and shape assessed by 3D photonic scanning. *International Journal of Body Composition Research, 8*, 123–130.

Stewart, A.D., Stewart, A. & Reid, D. (2002). Correcting calf circumference discriminates the incidence of falling but not bone quality by broadband ultrasound attenuation in elderly female subjects. *Bone, 31*, 195–198.

Tanaka, K. & Matsuura, Y. (1982). A multivariate analysis of the role of certain anthropometric and physiological attributes in distance running. *Annals of Human Biology, 9*, 473–482.

Taylor, R.W., Jones, I.E., Williams, S,M. & Goulding, A. (2000). Evaluation of waist circumference, waist-to-hip ratio, and the conicity index as screening tools for high trunk mass, as measured by dual-energy X-ray absorptiometry, in children 2–19 y. *American Journal of Clinical Nutrition, 72*, 490–495.

Tothill, P. & Stewart, A.D. (2002). Estimation of thigh muscle and adipose tissue volume using magnetic resonance imaging and anthropometry. *Journal of Sports Sciences, 20*, 563–576.

Tyrrell, A.R., Reilly, T. & Troup J.D.G. (1985). Circadian variation in stature and the effects of spinal loading. *Spine, 10*, 161–164.

Valdez, R. (1991). A simple model-based index of abdominal adiposity. *Journal of Clinical Epidemiology, 9*, 955–956.

Valsamakis, G., Chetty, R., Anwar, A., Banerjee, A.K., Barnett, A. & Kumar, S. (2004). Association of simple anthropometric measures of obesity with visceral fat and the metabolic syndrome. *Diabetic Medicine, 21*, 1339–1448.

van der Kooy, K., Leenen, R., Seidell, J.C., Deurenberg, P. & Visser, M. (1993). Abdominal diameters as indicators of visceral fat: comparison between magnetic resonance imaging and anthropometry. *British Journal of Nutrition, 70*, 47–58.

Vijayarghavan, K. & Gowrinath Sastry, J. (1976). The efficacy of arm circumference as a substitute for weight in assessment of protein-calorie malnutrition. *Annals of Human Biology, 3*, 229–233.

Wang, J., Thornton, J.C., Bari, S., Williamson, B., Gallagher, D., Heymsfield, S.B. et al. (2003). Comparisons of waist circumferences measured at 4 sites. *American Journal of Clinical Nutrition, 77*, 379–384.

WHO (World Health Organization). (2004). Appropriate body-mass index for Asian populations and its implications for policy and intervention strategies. *The Lancet, 363*, 157–163.

Yusuf, S., Hawken, S., Ôunpuu, S., Dans, T., Avezum, A., Lanas, F. et al. on behalf of the INTERHEART study investigators. (2004). Effect of potentially modifiable risk factors associated with myocardial infarction in 52 countries (the INTERHEART study): case-control study. *The Lancet, 364*, 937–952.

8

BODY COMPOSITION CHANGE

Patria A. Hume and Arthur D. Stewart

This chapter will cover:

8.1 Body composition changes associated with childhood, adolescence and adulthood from a health context
8.2 Childhood body composition, adolescent growth and health implications
8.3 Adult morphology and age-related body composition changes
8.4 Optimal size and proportions for ideal sport performance (morphological optimisation)
8.5 Tailoring soft tissue for maximum functional effectiveness (morphological prototype) in sport
8.6 Anticipating adult morphology in the growing child (morphological prediction) and implications for sports performance
8.7 Athlete talent identification and development for sports performance

8.1 Body composition changes associated with childhood, adolescence and adulthood from a health context

Humans differ from most other animals by having a fairly long lifespan and, proportionately, a long period of growth before adult morphology is attained. This chapter considers body composition changes associated with childhood, adolescence and adulthood from a health perspective, before considering in more detail how body composition can be adjusted in the context of sport. Although this might sound straightforward, consider that it might take 12 years of sports participation before a world class athlete attains a career best. Future capability needs to be recognised, understood and nurtured during childhood, while maintaining present health and safeguarding future health. Excessive training perturbs the body's homeostasis in musculo-skeletal, metabolic, endocrine, immune and psychological domains; however, it appears that individual tolerance of high exercise volume and susceptibility to overtraining is highly variable. Variability in the tempo of maturation in children can represent an advantage or disadvantage depending on the sport and gender. Knowledge of these issues is important for exercise practitioners and coaches alike, given the growing number of people whose body composition either predisposes them to increased risk of disease, or requires their body composition to be optimised in order to enhance performance and reduce injury risk. In this chapter we consider how kinanthropometry can be useful in youth sports for talent development and improving sports performance. We will explore the relationship between structure (as measured by anthropometry), physiology, psychology and skill for talent identification and how using these factors in isolation may risk overlooking potential champion athletes. We outline how to predict adult size and proportions from the growing child (morphological prediction), the optimal size and proportions for the ideal sports performance (morphological optimisation) in sport, and how athletes can tailor soft tissue for maximum functional effectiveness by training, tapering, etc. (morphological prototype). In addition, we examine how performance might be enhanced or retarded by biological maturity and how biological maturity is affected by energy balance in the young athlete.

The assessment of body composition for health has taken on greater significance because of the worrying increase in the global prevalence of obesity, and its related morbidity and mortality. The consequences of obesity are not only manifest in the diminished quality of life, but are felt acutely in the associated healthcare costs. Despite research efforts to understand the aetiology and molecular mechanisms associated with obesity making considerable advances, the implementation of lifestyle change at the population level has largely failed, so the trends we observe today are likely to continue, increasing the global burden of obesity in the future. This reality mandates a number of important research priorities relating to lifestyle and behaviours as well as many within the domain of body composition itself. These research priorities include the need to document and understand the tracking and heritability of body fatness, the need to relate fat patterning in childhood and fat patterning in adults, to link the changes in the prevalence of obesity in order to predict disease prevalence, mortality and healthcare costs, and to quantify the protective role of exercise on health in an integrated way using a life-span approach. Although it has been recognised that the development of physical fitness is protective over general health, culminating in the term 'health-related fitness' (Lohman, 1989), what is required is a strategic approach to quantify the dose-response of exercise for enhancing different physiological parameters such as blood pressure, insulin resistance, lipid profile etc. and provide culturally specific exercise advice matched to developmental stage.

In considering the lifespan stages we need to define key terms we will use in this chapter. *Growth* refers to the increase in size of a biological organism and typically characterises the first two decades of life in humans. Growth is largely under genetic control but is subject to environmental modification. Growth is non-uniform and takes place in discrete episodes. A phase of relatively rapid growth (referred to as saltation) may be followed by one of little or no relative growth (referred to as stasis). Growth is achieved as a result of a series of increments. There is non-uniformity of the tempo and timing of body tissues and systems undergoing growth. *Biological maturation* is the tempo and timing of progress towards the mature biological state (Malina, Bouchard & Bar-Or, 2004). *Somatic growth* is the progress towards adult stature, and considers only dimensional measurements. Size itself is a poor indictor of maturation in the absence of other data, such as parental stature. *Skeletal maturation* tracks the developing skeleton as it becomes mineralised, bone centres as they alter juxtaposition and epiphyseal plates as they grow and fuse (as discussed in Chapter 6). *Sexual maturation* represents the progress towards a mature biological state of full reproductive capability (ova production in girls and sperm production in boys) and is characterised by secondary sex characteristics such as genitalia and breast development, pubic and axillary hair growth, menarche in girls, and alteration in voice characteristics and facial hair in boys. *Sexual dimorphism* is where males and females exhibit a divergence in morphology which becomes more emphasised during adolescence.

8.2 Childhood body composition, adolescent growth and health implications

Childhood refers to the post infancy stage (after one year of age) leading up to adolescence. Some authors include a 'juvenile' stage before adolescence during which children can survive independently of parents, however in the present chapter this is considered as part of the childhood stage. Growth hormone and thyroid hormone are essential for growth. Growth hormone facilitates protein synthesis and mediates the proliferation of cartilage cells at the epiphyseal boundary which promotes somatic growth. Thyroid hormone promotes growth of the central nervous system and works in conjunction with growth hormone in stimulating bone and cartilage formation. Insulin-like growth factor is influential in protein synthesis and muscle growth. Normal growth can be undermined by nutritional deficiency, impairment of hormone production, or both.

Several markers of somatic growth are typically used to track children to adolescence. The velocity curves for stature and mass depict a rapid deceleration of growth in early childhood until three years of age when stature deceleration is reduced and the rate of weight gain begins to increase. Alteration in the relative quantities of fat during childhood is viewed as a health risk factor later in life. Rolland-Cachera et al. (1984) identified the adiposity rebound as the rise in body mass index after it reaches a nadir around age five or six, and related the corresponding age and the magnitude of the effect to later disease. While the inadequacy of body mass index (BMI) to assess composition has been addressed in previous chapters, there appears to be evidence of such a link. However, due to the inability of younger children to tolerate measurement procedures, assessments of stature and mass (and hence BMI) are prone to error, and data need to be interpreted with caution.

The growth rate in infancy exceeds that of the adolescent growth spurt. Less widely recognised is the mid-growth spurt typically occurring between 6.5 and 8.5 years, which is much smaller and less marked. Importantly, the capacity to detect the mid-growth spurt is limited by measurement frequency and measurement precision. Many children might only be measured annually, in which case the mid-growth spurt is unlikely to be detected. Precision error of measurements must be sufficiently small, so the modest effect of this spurt is not masked by the error of measurement. The adolescent growth spurt, later and more marked in boys, is more apparent and easily detected (typical values are illustrated in Figure 8.1). The observed adult difference in stature is mostly because boys grow approximately 5 cm per year for two extra years before commencing their growth spurt.

Growth charts have been in routine use since the late 1950s, but are not as straightforward to apply as they might seem, as highlighted by the review of Cameron (2002). The secular trend for increased stature of between 0.5 and 1.5 cm per decade reported during the 1970s appeared to have ceased by 1980. The validity of this or other secular trends is contingent on the similarity in morphology of the source data to those under investigation, and the sample size reflecting population parameters of ethnic variation and socio-economic status. Consideration is required of source data for growth charts because cross-sectional growth data, while useful in some respects, cannot illustrate normal growth variation in the timing and duration of the growth spurt (Cameron, 2002). The diagnosis of a growth disorder might be affected by which chart is used, which highlights the importance of standardisation of approach and the use of currently validated methods.

Adolescence refers to the phase of growth leading from puberty to adulthood by attaining structural and functional maturity. Puberty commences with increasing complexity and interaction of hormonal influence (growth hormone, insulin-like

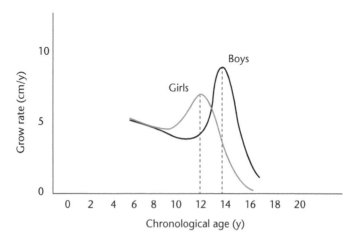

FIGURE 8.1 The adolescent growth spurt in girls and boys.

growth factor, thyroid hormone and cortisol, in addition to testosterone in boys and oestrogen in girls). Hormones largely determine the tissue mass gained during adolescence – mainly muscle in boys and fat (and also muscle) in girls. Also, during adolescence bone mineral gain is greater than its subsequent loss in later life after it typically peaks around age 30. Because up to 40 per cent of the variation in peak bone mass is considered to be modifiable by environmental factors, exposure to adequate high impact exercise and calcium intake during adolescence is essential to acquire a high peak value, and safeguard against osteopoenia and osteoporosis in later life. Somatic growth, manifesting in peak height velocity, typically displays a two-year difference between boys and girls. Since the 1950s there has been a secular trend for a reduction in the age at which peak height velocity occurs in both boys and girls. The gain in body mass also exhibits a similar profile, with males showing the same time lag, relative to females. However, different body tissues experience differential growth. For example an average healthy boy of 14 years might achieve 91 per cent of his adult stature but only 72 per cent of his adult muscle mass, and only by 18 years will muscle mass rise to 91 per cent, when stature growth might be approaching zero (Buckler, 1990).

Adolescence is probably most known for the sexual maturation that occurs during this phase of development. The progression through adolescence has been intensively investigated by Tanner and colleagues, and the five stages of sexual maturation, known as 'Tanner stages' which rate the secondary sex characteristics of an individual have been ubiquitously applied to growth studies for over half a century. Due to the invasive nature of clinical examination of genitalia and pubic hair development, such routine tests which were performed in schools are now rare. Instead, different approaches can be used to rate maturity, including children self-rating, parental rating, or using other morphological characteristics such as peak height velocity.

The assessment of body composition in children has taken on greater significance because of the likelihood of obese children becoming obese adults, and that lifestyle behaviours acquired in childhood are resistant to change. While our understanding of aetiology of childhood obesity remains incomplete, several factors have a direct or indirect influence over energy intake or expenditure. Higher body fat content is associated with early maturation in girls (early menarche) and greater fat acquisition throughout adolescence. The effect of body fat content on maturation is less well established in boys, possibly as a result of the rapid increase in muscle mass that typifies growth in adolescent boys. Earlier sexual maturation in girls, relative to boys, means that physical activity is de-emphasised, commonly in favour of social activity. While performance capability of boys may exceed that of girls, the importance of maintaining physical activity in terms of health can be argued to be of greater importance for girls. Increasing energy expenditure via exercise can help reduce fat while fat-free mass is maintained. However, assessment of change in fat mass and fat-free mass needs to take into account the instability of fat-free mass during the growth and developmental processes (Boileau, Lohman and Slaughter, 1985), which is rarely appreciated.

A number of studies have assessed changes in anthropometric characteristics of children such as Corroll's (1986) study of Manitoba children aged 6 to 18 years between 1967 and 1980, and Kondric's (Kondric & Misigoj-Durakovic, 2002) study of 2,372 Slovenian primary and secondary male students aged 7 to 18 years. The implementation of an individualised approach to physical education curriculum development due to variability of morphological development and varying levels of motor ability has been recommended (Kondric & Misigoj-Durakovic, 2002). The 'Healthy Hearts' longitudinal study of cardio-metabolic health in 902 youth aged 6 to 15 years (McGavock, Torrance, McGuire, Wozny & Lewanczuk, 2009) showed that children with low cardio-respiratory fitness were characterised by larger waist circumference and disproportionate weight gain over a 12-month follow-up period.

8.3 Adult morphology and age-related body composition changes

The stages of young adulthood (age 18–24 years), adulthood (25–44 years), middle age (45–64 years) and subsequently old age (Spirduso, 1995) involve anatomical and functional changes which tend to optimise functional capacity in young adulthood, after which it declines. The primary tissues of the skeletal system and muscular system as well as adipose tissue all follow a trajectory in adulthood that is the function of the interaction between genetic, hormonal and environmental interaction. Skeletal size and shape are configured earlier in this trajectory than bone density (bone tissue is considered in detail in Chapter 6). After peak height velocity is attained in the adolescent growth spurt, stature declines to zero growth, although incremental growth in skeletal breadth (e.g. biacromial breadth and bicristal breadth) and chest depth commonly continue after the adolescent growth spurt. Final stature does not indicate the skeletal shape or peak bone density is finalised. Significant height (commonly up to 8 cm) may be lost in adulthood and old age as a result of postural changes and structural alterations in the spine caused by osteoporosis. Weight-bearing exercise in adulthood generally maintains or reduces the rate of loss of bone, rather than adding bone. Studies of the elderly may enquire of participants' stature at age 25 years or alternatively measure the height of the tibial plateau from the standing surface while the participant is standing. In addition, chest depth enlarges as a result of loss of compliance of the thorax.

During young adulthood, muscle mass tends to accumulate although the extent of its accrual depends on activity and interaction between genetic factors and environmental factors (muscle tissue is considered in Chapter 5). The widely recognised decline in fat-free mass commencing in adulthood until old age tends to be primarily the loss of muscle tissue, related to the decline in growth hormone. Loss of muscle mass has been estimated to be 3 kg per decade on average in sedentary individuals (Forbes & Reina, 1970), with males losing approximately 1.5 times that of females. Exercise can reduce the rate of muscle loss by about 25 per cent (Buskirk & Hodgson, 1987). Muscles in regular use experience less atrophy, and the regeneration of muscle tends to replace slow twitch fibres more than fast twitch fibres, with the effect that slower less forceful muscle action is facilitated. In parallel, vestibular and visual deficits, gait deviations and loss of motor control all conspire against the functional mobility of the elderly, with the inevitable consequence of loss of confidence and increased risk of falls. Regular physical activity can provide a range of cues across these domains, perpetuating functional independence.

Adipose tissue tends to be gained systematically in both males and females during adulthood. Observations of fat patterning, and the typically android and gynoid shapes attributed to its distribution are well established. Males accumulate more visceral fat than women and tend to accumulate fat on the torso, while females accumulate fat in the gluto-femoral region. Gluto-femoral deposition of fat appears to be protective of health if it offers an alternative depot for excess fat. After menopause, females show signs of increased centralisation of excess fat to the torso, including both the subcutaneous and visceral depots. While muscle tissue obeys the law of specificity, in terms of use and retention, it does not recruit fat stores locally, so the concept of 'spot reduction' of fat stores is unfounded. Interventions which reduce overall body fat will tend to reduce all depots of fat, and not neglect one depot in favour of others. There appears to be no 'iceberg principle' by which the proportion of subcutaneous and visceral fat are in proportion, as was illustrated in a study of liposuction where obese women showed no reduction in visceral fat after removal of 71 of subcutaneous adipose tissue (Klein et al., 2004). While epidemiological evidence points to visceral fat being the primary 'health harming' fat, there are many variations which are worth noting. The 'fit-fat' distribution (as mentioned in Chapter 1) is where prolonged structured exercise preferentially utilises abdominal adipose tissue, under conditions of energy deficit or energy balance. Guidelines aimed at the general population by the US Department of Agriculture recommend that individuals engage in moderate to vigorous intensity activity on most days per week, while not exceeding caloric requirements. This advice was tested in a 12-month randomised control trial of sedentary individuals (McTiernan et al., 2007) with modest, though significant reductions in weight, BMI, waist circumference and body fat (assessed by dual X-ray absorptiometry). Exercisers who attained a greater number of steps per day (measured by pedometer) or greater exercise time also had greater reductions in weight, body mass index, total fat and intra-abdominal fat. The evidence points towards the effect of exercise preferentially utilising abdominal fat in previously sedentary individuals. Increased exercise can add muscle mass while at the same time reducing fat mass with the result that weight change is minimal. Individuals with only a small reduction in weight can therefore be healthier in terms of risk profile via a range of cardiorespiratory, metabolic and neuromuscular factors, and have greater functional capacity as a result of adaptation to exercise. Many studies of the efficacy of dietary interventions consider weight loss or change in body mass index as the outcome variable usually because they are easily measured, and have large comparative data sets available, even though body composition measurement would be more valid.

We need to be mindful of how to interpret the trajectory of body composition change in adulthood. As a person ages, the probability of death increases, and the mean survival age is less than the mean life expectancy in the absence of premature death. The ageing population is increasingly highly selected so our interpretation of morphological changes needs to take this into account. Morbidity pervades an increasing number of elderly individuals, largely as a result of the capabilities of modern medicine to prolong life and slow disease progression. These factors are important when considering cross-sectional data, which typically form the evidence base for the study of ageing. Secular trends in life expectancy have shown changes in body composition in later life being the consequence of a health disorder which may at some future point prove fatal. For example, approximately 30 per cent of Americans 60–69 years have no chronic health conditions, but the percentage with no chronic health conditions reduces to 10 per cent in adults 80 years and over. The shape of curves for body weight, body mass index or total fat against age decline in old age, reflecting the preferential survival of less overweight individuals.

An approach of functional health associated with advancing years has used masters athletes to quantify the scope for retaining physical capabilities. Although body composition data are not available, and there are assumptions regarding performance optimisation, observation of masters athletes' performance relative to historic records can quantify a range of physiological factors that have enhanced our understanding of the training process. Ageing muscle favours slow twitch activity and generally exhibits less hypertrophy in response to specific training stimuli. While intensity and volume of training tends be reduced in masters athletes, relative to elite young adult athletes, recent evidence points to reduced regenerative capacity following muscle damage. Although young and old muscles are equally prone to damage, there appears to be greater sensitivity to modest levels of damage in older muscle tissue (Thalacker-Mercer, Dell'Italia, Cui, Cross & Bamman, 2010) which is important in a range of settings. Masters athletes require longer recovery relative to younger athletes as the vulnerability for elderly muscles to damage diminishes the consequent exercise load in a self-limiting manner. Elderly individuals undergoing surgery may be unable to restore the affected muscle mass to pre-surgery levels despite intensive physical intervention.

Taken together, the body composition changes during adulthood are complex and closely related to functional changes. The scope to continue activity that slows the age-related changes in body composition and functional capacity is wide, although individuals generally experience diminishing athletic horizons with age, exacerbated by a range of medical conditions. While some conditions such as type-2 diabetes may be the result of adverse body composition, others, such as osteoarthritis may result from accumulated wear and tear, and a reduced capacity for regeneration. Today, the scope for survival with impaired health has never been greater. As a consequence, the limits of the variability of human body composition are being extended as living adults may survive below 30 kg in severe undernourishment and exceed 600 kg in extreme obesity.

8.4 Optimal size and proportions for ideal sport performance (morphological optimisation)

Sports performance generally involves maximising force, acceleration, speed or mechanical efficiency. In fulfilment of these biomechanical imperatives, there are optimal size and proportions underpinning the ideal performance in sport, referred to as *morphological optimisation*. Some sports have morphology-related limiting factors that prevent players from reaching elite levels (e.g. gymnastics, weight lifting, court sports and contact sports), while other sports seem to have few morphology-related limiting factors (e.g. racquet sports, mobile field sports, and set field sports).

Morphology-related limiting factors are prevalent in elite competitors in gymnastics, diving and power sports, where performance may be limited by angular acceleration. Gymnasts and divers are typically the smallest and lightest of all sports people, with a high ratio of sitting height to stature caused by shorter than average lower limb lengths (see Figure 8.2A). Historically, world class performances have been achieved in these sports in children still to attain adult stature. Weight lifters and power lifters have a high ratio of sitting height to stature caused by shorter than average upper and lower limb lengths, as well as low crural and brachial indexes (i.e. a short distal segment of the lower and upper limb, respectively) (see Figure 8.2B). Distance runners are short and light athletes with relatively short lower limbs and a high crural index (tibia : femur length) and a low brachial (radius : humerus length) index.

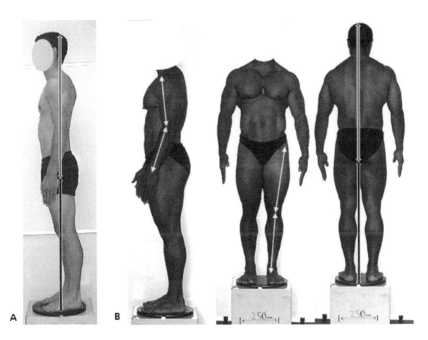

FIGURE 8.2 Gymnasts (A) and power lifters (B) typically have a high ratio of sitting height to stature caused by shorter than average lower limb lengths. Power lifters also typically have a low crural index (tibia/thigh) and low brachial index (forearm/upper arm).

A low skelic index appears characteristic of female strength athletes while a low brachial index is typical of female endurance and strength athletes. These findings are congruent with biomechanical imperatives to maximise force and/or minimise energy expenditure offering sports-specific advantage (Stewart et al., 2010). In athletic field events such as discus and javelin, competitors are generally tall and possess a high brachial index. Jumpers have a high relative lower limb length and a high crural index that provide a mechanically advantageous lever system for jumping. Court sports such as basketball, netball and volleyball have athletes that rely on jumping prowess and must have a linear physique and a high relative lower limb length. These athletes typically have a low ratio of sitting height to stature caused by longer than average lower limb lengths. These ratios vary significantly according to team position (e.g. in basketball players). Contact field sports such as rugby and football are affected by body size with several specialist positions requiring tall stature and increased body mass, where absolute rather than relative power is paramount. Several morphology-related limiting factors exist for aquatic sports. Elite sprint and slalom paddlers generally possess a high brachial index, which delivers greater leverage. World championship performance in swimming is influenced by tall stature and absolute limb lengths as well as the size of hands and feet. Tall, linear physiques provide some advantage for tennis players on certain playing surfaces, but smaller, more agile players can be more successful on a slower clay court surface. Taller physiques are also an advantage for fast bowlers in cricket to increase the lever length in ball delivery. Such physiques may also be an advantage for soccer players in certain playing positions such as in goal-scoring opportunities from a goal kick, while smaller, more agile soccer players tend to be more successful in other roles. Combative sports vary in their ideal physiques, by counterpoising the advantage offered by reach and a linear morphology (as in tae kwon do) with that offered by a low centre of mass and consequent stability of a broader physique (as in wrestling and judo) (Ackland, Kerr & Newton, 2009). Taken together, these structural advantages offered by skeletal factors that do not respond to athletic training have implications for selectivity of sports in which athletes are likely to excel. Structural disadvantages do not preclude success but require that some physiological or psychological factor to negate the disadvantage resulting from morphological factors. Knowledge of the morphology-related limiting factors can be useful for selection criteria for youth athletes when entering a sport, as long as the measurements are stable during youth and adolescence, or valid prediction methods are available based on sound research including longitudinal data analyses.

8.5 Tailoring soft tissue for maximum functional effectiveness (morphological prototype) in sport

With the essential skeletal framework largely determined genetically, how can athletes fine tune the physique for optimal performance? Bodily tissues can be theoretically grouped as 'active' or 'ballast' whether they enhance or retard force generation. Extra muscle for strength must be 'worth its own weight', and relative strength has been shown to scale to mass raised to the power 0.69, with composition assumed to be constant. Some muscle groups are rate-limiters for force production while others are merely passive. Altering strength in one muscle group alters length-tension relationships and inertial properties, and may destabilise joints and lead to injury. With current emphasis on core stability for several sports, in others, such as flat racing or time trial cycling, adding mass to the upper body may be considered a disadvantage.

In contrast to the law of specificity of training affecting muscle, adipose tissue responds to the body's energy balance in a more general way. Excess adipose tissue stored as an energy surplus will adversely affect performance in most sports. However, viewed as an endocrine organ responsible for the production of bio-molecules implicated in our general health, we should be careful to ensure the athlete's health (and in female athletes, specifically reproductive health) is not threatened as a result of training that seeks to optimise sports performance. An athlete's physique responds to the periodisation in a training programme in a dynamic way, by adjusting adipose tissue, muscle tissue, glycogen stores and water balance. This phenomenon was first described in relation to the proximity to Olympic competition in ice skaters as *morphological prototype*. Anthropometric tools have been used in profiling athletes' trajectory thereby optimising the trainable parameters at the times which they mattered most. This has important implications for weight category sports, where athletes may be at risk of employing unsafe weight control practices in order to 'make weight'.

The issue for establishing minimum weight is one of the most pertinent and problematic affecting today's athletes. As the pressure to excel advances in parallel to standards of athletic achievement, athletes and coaches consider every conceivable means of enhancing performance. There has been abuse of drugs, which clouded the weight lifting events of the 1970s and the professional cycling circuit in the 1990s, to enforced dehydration in order to reduce body weight below the target in sports such as weight lifting and rowing. Where the health of the athlete is concerned, especially for junior athletes, legislation may be essential in order to safeguard health, yet some bizarre and health-harming practices prevail. In response to the tragic death of American college wrestlers in 1997, research was conducted in various laboratories across several US states to establish criteria for minimum body weight in wrestling, and to inform weight control programmes which were applied across several states as a result. However, the practice of weight 'cutting' (rapid weight loss prior to competition) still appears to be widespread, and has been previously demonstrated to threaten health and normal growth (Convertino et al., 1996). The American College of Sports Medicine's exercise and fluid replacement position stand is well considered, but lacking federal authority as it requires individual states to voluntarily accept the suggested weight control practices.

An International Olympic Committee Medical Commission working group on body composition was commissioned in 2010 to investigate how to protect the health of athletes. It identified three categories of sports that represent a health risk:

gravitational sports, weight category sports and aesthetic sports. Gravitational sports involve the body working in a vertical plane by applying forces to overcome gravity, such as endurance running, cycling and ski jumping. Weight category sports include all types of combative sport such as judo and tae kwon do, as well as rowing and weightlifting. Aesthetic sports involve appearance, poise and highly skilled body movements such as figure skating, gymnastics and diving. All these sports share a common influence of the pressure for leanness, minimising fat levels and optimising power-to-weight ratio. For example, in the mid-1990s, the rules for ski jumping were altered due to the flight advantage of very lean and slender individuals, whose body composition represented a performance advantage, but a health risk (Müller, 2009). While the International Olympic Committee lacks authority to implement rules outside the Olympics, they do have a world stage for sharing best practice, and where necessary can help alter rules where there is a clear mandate to do so.

8.6 Anticipating adult morphology in the growing child (morphological prediction) and implications for sports performance

We have considered factors that prevail concerning adult performance, each exerting its independent influence, so now we consider factors affecting morphology and the potential for growth at any time point before adulthood. This is not straightforward as there needs to be consideration of predicting adult size, in addition to biological maturation, each with consequences for performance.

Skeletal age assessment, which is perhaps the most reliable of maturation indices, incurs X-ray exposure and ethical issues. Assessment of secondary sex characteristics is considered intrusive and self-assessment may be unreliable, and serial measurements of stature required to identify peak height velocity may not be possible or valid. Although females generally mature earlier than males, large individual variability confounds easy prediction of final stature. A viable alternative involves a validated equation by Mirwald, Baxter-Jones, Bailey & Beunen (2002) based on the mean peak height velocity (~13.45 years in boys and ~11.77 years in girls in their sample) and its relation to sitting height and leg length and their interaction. A maturity offset regression predicts the time from peak height velocity in cross-validated gender-specific regression models, so final stature can be anticipated, knowing the likelihood of the remaining growth trajectory. Such an estimate can then be coupled with morphological optimisation prospectively in talent identification.

Sexual maturation affects morphology and sports performance. In school sports settings, early maturers may excel in team sports as a result of size and speed advantages, and sexual dimorphism alters the power-to-weight ratio during adolescence positively in males and usually negatively in females, with consequences for power sports. Because it may take four or more years for 95 per cent of children to pass the same maturation 'milestone' the process may disguise athletic talent,

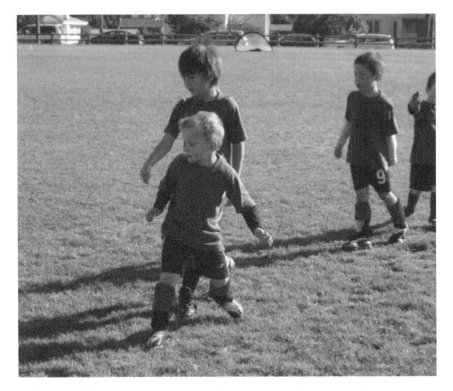

FIGURE 8.3 Differences in stature even at five years can affect sport performance.

with the result that early maturing females and late maturing males are easily overlooked. However, variability in somatic growth is manifest much earlier than adolescence. There can be large differences in stature even at five years which can affect sport performance (see Figure 8.3).

8.7 Athlete talent identification and development for sports performance

Talent *identification* describes the scientific process used to identify talent. Talent *detection* is the process used to identify talent from outside the sport and talent *selection* allows the identification of talent from within the sport. Talent *development* is where those with identified talent are provided with opportunity to achieve full potential. Kinanthropometry can be useful in youth sports for talent detection, selection and development programmes.

There are a number of challenges facing talent identification in sport:

A   talent identification has a morphological component, whose influence varies between sports and individuals, depending on a range of other factors such as skill;

B   morphological optimisation concerns the non-trainable skeletal factors which can advantage/disadvantage an individual in certain sports;

C   morphological prototype concerns the soft tissue (muscle and adipose) which creates and partly retards movement but also has influence over general health; and

D   the overlapping of these three factors is complicated and we must also consider biological growth and maturation which profoundly influence performance, differently in girls and boys, and differently again between sports and fast or slow maturers (see Figure 8.4).

The key to unravelling this complex web of interdependent influences is to start with reliable measures which are allied to sports performance.

Often in an attempt to determine anthropometric characteristics that may be useful for screening youth athletes, comparisons are made between youth and elite athletes, or athlete and non-athletes. For example, morphological analyses of six female and 18 male youth tennis players compared to their non-sport peers showed that the majority of youth tennis players were taller, had longer lower limbs and lower amounts of adipose tissue and larger arm circumferences compared to their non-sport peers (Bojzan, Pietraszewska, Migasiewicz, Tomaszewski, & Bach, 2008). Prediction functions have been developed for the best variables that distinguish between talented and less talented team sports players aged 11 to 16

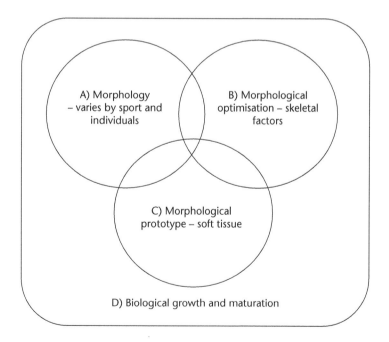

FIGURE 8.4 Morphology challenges facing talent identification in sport.

years in rugby, soccer, field hockey and netball (Spamer & Coetzee, 2002). While these types of comparisons are useful in tracking youths towards elite performance, the individual variability in growth, the lack of stability of measures throughout adolescence, and the limited predictability of performance from unidimensional data, means that their utility is limited.

Sports performance can be enhanced or retarded by biological maturity. Biological maturity is affected by energy balance in the young athlete delaying maturation in some groups. Early maturers are often taller, heavier, more powerful and faster than their counterparts during the early to mid-teenage years, which has often led to selection biases in sporting competitions grouped by chronological age. Anderson & Ward (2002) proposed a classification system for youth sports that is maturation-based, using the anthropometric prediction of vertical jump impulse potential. Impulse was calculated for children between 8 to 18 years from vertical jump height ($I = m[2gh]^{0.5}$). Equations were developed that accounted for differences in muscle tissue development while utilising variables easily measured in both males and females, including chronological age and measures of height, forearm girth and calf girth. Using restricted ranges of impulse scores, males and females could be classed into appropriate groups for competition and sport, competing together until the age of 14. At and beyond this age, females had a similar capacity to generate impulse and could compete in one group, while restricted impulse categories could be useful for males until the age of 18 years.

Coelho e Silva, Figueiredo & Malina (2003) assessed physical growth and maturation related variation in 112 Portuguese young male soccer players. The effect of chronological age on body size was evident within the 11–12 year group and 13–14 year group, while the effect of maturational status on motor performance was only significant within the older group. The reduced variation in older boys reflects approaching maturity in late adolescence. Hirose (2009) examined physical and maturational differences between 332 adolescent elite soccer players who were considered to have high potential to play soccer at a professional level as decided subjectively by coaches. There was a bias according to quarter of year of birth which depended on differences in individual skeletal age and body size. The height of players born in the last quarter of the year was significantly smaller than those of players born in the first quarter of the year when data were adjusted for maturation. Hirose recommended that individual biological maturation should be considered when selecting adolescent soccer players.

Caution is advised when attempting to predict future adult sport performances based on adolescent testing because of the varied stability of physical traits during adolescent growth. Segment breadths remain relatively stable throughout adolescence and can be used for predictive purposes, however, segment lengths are usually unstable and should not be used as prediction criteria for talent identification. Segment length variability (e.g. a six per cent change in leg length to sitting height ratio) can form the basis for a final stature prediction based on the maturity offset (Mirwald et al., 2002). The accuracy of body composition measurements must also be taken into account when tracking athletes over time (Hume & Marfell-Jones, 2008).

Changing morphology of the growing athlete and the skill level acquired are inevitably interlinked, so models that combine dimensional measures with skill are warranted. A multidisciplinary selection model for youth soccer was developed by Vaeyens et al. (2006) based on analyses of relationships between physical (anthropometry and maturity status), sport-specific performance characteristics and level of skill in elite, sub-elite, and non-elite youth soccer players in four age groups between 12–16 years. Characteristics that discriminated successful youth soccer players varied with competitive age levels. Talent identification models should be flexible and provide opportunities for changing parameters in a long-term developmental context.

Complex and dynamic interrelationships between anatomical structure, physiology, psychology and skill prevail in sport. If any of these factors is used for talent identification in isolation there is a risk of overlooking potential winners, a finding which the scientific and coaching communities have been slow to appreciate. A range of relevant anthropometric factors can be considered which are subject to strong genetic influences (e.g. stature), or are largely environmentally determined and susceptible to training effects. Consequently, anthropometric profiling can generate a useful database against which talented groups may be compared. There have been several major sport studies conducted at Olympic Games starting with the Amsterdam Olympics in 1928, and at world championships for sports such as swimming and football. However, anthropometric measurement alone does not provide a representative assessment of a player's physical capabilities in sports where open skills are influential. There may be marked individual differences in anthropometric and physiological characteristics among elite performers. For example, top-class soccer players have to adapt to the physical demands of the game, which are multi-factorial. Players may not need to have an extraordinary capacity within any of the areas of physical performance, but must possess a reasonably high level within all areas (Reilly, Bangsbo & Franks, 2000).

Assessing body composition in the growing and developing individual is fraught with difficulty because of a range of issues. Increasing energy expenditure can reduce fat while fat-free body mass can be maintained. However, the dual metabolic challenges of exercise and growth deplete the same reserve, violating methodological assumptions concerning stability of the fat-free body mass and rendering change detection problematic. Even though a range of methods suitable for children is available, including anthropometry and body density, accuracy in predicting fat mass and fat-free mass can be poorer than assumed. Individual variability is such that the threshold of performance impairment due to chronic depletion of energy reserves will tend to differ between individuals. In this context, the pragmatic solution is to align anthropometric data with those of performance, fatigue and general health. Coaches are best placed to do this after a full dialogue with both the athlete and the sports scientist.

Summary

The scope for body composition change throughout life (childhood, adolescence and adulthood) from a health context is vast. The physique trajectory which has both genetic and environmental determinants can be anticipated up to a point, for identifying disease or sporting talent. Body composition can be adjusted in the context of sport by tailoring soft tissue for maximum functional effectiveness. The nature of talent identification is holistic so coaches need to consider not only performance, skill and psychological factors, but also anthropometric factors that are growth-related, training-related and that anticipate adult morphology. There must be care in predicting future adult performances based on adolescent testing because of the varied stability of physical traits during growth. Segment breadths remain stable in relation to stature throughout adolescence and can be used for predictive purposes, however segment lengths are unstable and should not be used as prediction criteria in talent identification programmes. Proportionality can be an important self-selector for sports. Alignment of morphology to performance, and recognition of the wide individual variability in maturation rate, will help avoid biasing athlete selection, or overlooking talented individuals with potential to excel. Early maturers are often taller, heavier, more powerful and faster than late maturers during the early to mid-teenage years, which has often led to selection biases in sporting competitions grouped by chronological age. Coaches need to consider anthropometric characteristics and changes over the lifespan to avoid biasing their athlete selection.

References

Ackland, T.R., Kerr, D.A. & Newton, R.U. (2009). Modifying physical capacities. In T.A. Ackland, B.C. Elliot & J. Bloomfield (Eds.). *Applied Anatomy and Biomechanics in Sport* (2nd edition, pp. 227–276). Champaign, IL: Human Kinetics.

Anderson, G.S. & Ward, R. (2002). Classifying children for sports participation based upon anthropometric measurement. *European Journal of Sport Science, 2*, 1–13.

Boileau, R.A., Lohman, T.G. & Slaughter, M.H. (1985). Exercise and body composition of children and youth. *Scandinavian Journal of Sports Sciences, 7*, 17–27.

Bojzan, A., Pietraszewska, J., Migasiewicz, J., Tomaszewski, W. & Bach, W. (2008). Selected anthropometric parameters of young tennis players in the context of the usefulness for this sports discipline and motor organ contusion prophylaxis. *Medycyna Sportowa, 24*, 337–347.

Buckler, J. (1990). *A Longitudinal Study of Adolescent Growth.* London: Springer-Verlag.

Buskirk, E.R. & Hodgson, J.L. (1987). Age and aerobic power: the rate of change in men and women. *Federation Proceedings, 46*, 1824–1829.

Cameron, N. (2002). British growth charts for height and weight with recommendations concerning their use in auxological assessment. *Annals of Human Biology, 29*, 1–10.

Coelho e Silva, M., Figueiredo, A. & Malina, R.M. (2003). Physical growth and maturation related variation in young male soccer athletes. *Acta Kinesiologiae Universitatis Tartuensis, 8*, 34–50.

Convertino, V.A., Armstrong, L.E., Coyle, E.F., Mack, G.W., Sawka, M.N., Senay Jr., L.C., et al. (1996). American College of Sports Medicine position stand: exercise and fluid replacement. *Medicine and Science in Sports and Exercise, 28*(1), i–vii.

Corroll, V. (1986). Status and changes of anthropometric and physical performance measures of Manitoba youth, 6 to 18 years of age, between 1967 and 1980. In J.A.P. Day (Ed.), *Perspectives in Kinanthropometry* (pp. 99–106). Champaign, IL: Human Kinetics Publishers.

Forbes, G.B. & Reina, J.C. (1970). Adult lean body mass declines with age: some longitudinal observations. *Metabolism, 19*, 653–663.

Hirose, N. (2009). Relationships among birth-month distribution, skeletal age and anthropometric characteristics in adolescent elite soccer players. *Journal of Sports Sciences, 27*, 1159–1166.

Hume, P.A. & Marfell-Jones, M. (2008). The importance of accurate site location in skinfold measurement. *Journal of Sport Sciences, 26*, 1333–1340.

Klein, S., Fontana, L., Young, L., Coggan, A. R., Kilo, C., Patterson, B.W. et al. (2004). Absence of an effect of liposuction on insulin action and risk factors for coronary heart disease. *New England Journal of Medicine, 350*, 2549–2557.

Kondric, M. & Misigoj-Durakovic, M. (2002). Changes of certain anthropometric characteristics in boys 7 to 18 years of age. *International Journal of Physical Education, 39*, 30–35.

Lohman, T.G. (1989). Assessment of body composition in children. *Pediatric Exercise Science, 1*, 19–30.

Malina, R.M., Bouchard, C. & Bar-Or, O. (2004). *Growth, Maturation and Physical Activity* (2nd edition). Champaign, IL: Human Kinetics.

McGavock, J.M., Torrance, B.D., McGuire, K.A., Wozny, P.D. & Lewanczuk, R.Z. (2009). Cardiorespiratory fitness and the risk of overweight in youth: the healthy hearts longitudinal study of cardiometabolic health. *Obesity, 17*, 1802–1807.

McTiernan, A., Sorensen, B., Irwin, M.L., Morgan, M., Yasui, Y., Rudolph, R.E. et al. (2007). Exercise effect on weight and body fat in men and women. *Obesity, 15*, 1496–1512.

Mirwald, R.L., Baxter-Jones, A.D.G., Bailey, D.A., & Beunen, G.P. (2002). An assessment of maturity from anthropometric measurements. *Medicine and Science in Sports and Exercise, 34*, 689–694.

Müller, W. (2009). Towards research-based approaches for solving body composition problems in sports: ski jumping as a heuristic example. *British Journal of Sports Medicine, 43*, 1013–1019.

Reilly, T., Bangsbo, J. & Franks, A. (2000). Anthropometric and physiological predispositions for elite soccer. *Journal of Sports Sciences, 18*, 669–683.

Rolland-Cachera, M.F., Deheeger, M., Bellisle, F., Semple, M., Guilloud-Bataille, M. & Patois, E. (1984). Adiposity rebound in children: a simple indicator for predicting obesity. *American Journal of Clinical Nutrition, 39*, 129–135.

Spamer, E.J. & Coetzee, M. (2002). Variables which distinguish between talented and less talented participants in youth sport – a comparative study. *Kinesiology, 34*, 141–152.

Spirduso, W.W. (1995). *Physical Dimensions of Aging*. Champaign, IL: Human Kinetics.

Stewart, A.D., Benson, P.J., Olds, T., Marfell-Jones, M., MacSween, A. & Nevill, A.M. (2010). Self selection of athletes into sports via skeletal ratios. In D.C. Lieberman (Ed.), *Aerobic Exercise and Athletic Performance: Types, Duration and Health Benefits*. New York: Nova Science Publishers.

Thalacker-Mercer, A.E., Dell'Italia, L.J., Cui, X., Cross, J.M. & Bamman, M.M. (2010). Differential genomic responses in old versus young humans despite similar levels of modest muscle damage after resistance loading. *Physiology Genomics, 40,* 141–149.

Vaeyens, R., Malina, R.M., Janssens, M., Van Renterghem, B., Bourgois, J., Vrijens, J. et al. (2006). A multidisciplinary selection model for youth soccer: the Ghent Youth Soccer Project. *British Journal of Sports Medicine, 40,* 928–934.

9

BODY COMPOSITION IN CHRONIC DISEASE AND DISABILITY

Vicky L. Goosey-Tolfrey and Laura Sutton

This chapter will cover:

9.1 Overview
9.2 Body composition in chronic disease
9.3 Consequences of physical disability
9.4 General considerations for the assessment of body composition

9.1 Overview

Body composition is labile and changes as a result of chronic disease, such as metabolic or wasting disorders, and disability. In addition to direct anatomical and physiological effects, the changes in lifestyle associated with such conditions also impact upon body composition. There is a growing interest to understand and evaluate the body composition of individuals with chronic diseases and disabilities. However, for these population groups special attention is warranted since the disease pathology, disability or treatment may alter the basic underlying body composition assumptions and measurement techniques that have been described previously.

The evaluation of body composition for normal healthy individuals across the exercise continuum is an important aspect of this book. Yet it is apparent that many equations used for assessment are considered population specific: the accuracy is dependent upon consideration of the population to be investigated. For example, generalised equations validated using predominantly Caucasian groups may lack accuracy in black populations, given the greater density of the fat-free mass (Schutte et al., 1984). As a further example, no standards for accurate assessment of percentage body fat exist for persons with a spinal cord injury (SCI), which limits the assessment of intervention programmes if fat loss is the desired goal. Due to the unique physiological consequences of SCI such as muscle atrophy, changes in tissue hydration and bone demineralisation, which vary according to the level and completeness of the SCI, violations of any underlying assumptions in methods of body composition analysis may be magnified substantially.

In subsequent sections the physiological and anatomical consequences of several specific chronic diseases and disabilities will be discussed, and the validity and reliability of methods of body composition analysis previously presented in this book will be considered with specific reference to disease and/or disability. It is beyond the scope of this chapter to discuss the associated body composition considerations for all chronic diseases and disabilities. Rather, it is designed to raise the awareness of these special population groups by using several specific chronic diseases and disabilities as a vehicle to enable the reader to understand how to apply their knowledge to a condition perhaps beyond their primary area of expertise.

9.2 Body composition in chronic disease

Changes in body composition may arise as a cause or consequence of disease, or indeed both. Body composition research has aided the understanding of many disease processes, and the monitoring of body composition is important in the clinical setting.

When considering body composition risk factors for disease, much of the focus tends to fall on the consequences of overweight and obesity, for example obese individuals are at greater risk of cardiovascular disease, certain cancers and diabetes mellitus. However, it should be borne in mind that underweight may also have causal links with disorders, for example, osteoporosis.

Changes in body composition may result as a consequence of diseases that alter physiological processes such as metabolism, psychological processes, or indirectly, for example through subsequent physical inactivity. In addition, the changes in body composition associated with a particular disease may result in an increased risk of additional health-related problems or disorders.

In the present section, an overview of some common conditions associated with altered body composition is presented. Disease groups considered include metabolic disorders, cardiovascular and pulmonary disease, wasting disorders and neuro-muscular disease.

9.2.1 Metabolic disease

Metabolic processes consist of sequences of chemical reactions that occur in living organisms in order to maintain life. Substances are broken down or built up through catabolic and anabolic processes, respectively, resulting in energy production and growth. Metabolic diseases are those associated with abnormalities in metabolism, i.e. disorders that alter metabolic processes and rate. Some metabolic diseases bring about changes in body composition; other disorders may occur, or increase in severity, as a side-effect of such changes.

Obesity

Obesity is a condition defined as 'abnormal or excessive fat accumulation in adipose tissue to the extent that health may be impaired' (Garrow, 1988; as cited in WHO, 2000, p.6). Definitions of obesity based on the body mass index are provided in Table 9.1. Often described as an epidemic, levels of obesity continue to be of concern in the developed world. Whilst the ability to store fat has aided the survival of the human race in the past (providing insulation from cold temperatures, protection for the internal organs and a source of reserve energy), today in the developed world the surplus availability of food and the increased automation of society allow an imbalance between energy intake and expenditure to occur, causing secular trends of rising obesity.

Further to the amount of excess body fat, the distribution, or 'fat patterning', is of importance, as certain depots, such as visceral adiposity, are associated with a higher risk of obesity-related diseases (Kissebah & Krakower, 1994). The increasing prevalence of overweight and obesity is associated with higher incidence of a number of diseases such as diabetes mellitus, coronary heart disease and cancer.

As a consequence of high body mass, bone mineral density is often above average in obese individuals, due to skeletal loading. Muscle mass may also be increased, as a means to support the excess weight. However, once obesity develops to a point at which physical activity is impeded, or as obese patients age, muscle mass is generally lost and bone mineral density may decrease. Expected tissue hydration is similar to non-obese values, but there may be greater variation within obesity groups.

TABLE 9.1 Risk of adverse health consequences for adults based on body mass index classifications

	BMI	Risk
Underweight	<18.5	Low
Normal	18.5–24.9	Average
Overweight	≥25.0	Increased
Preobese	25.0–29.9	Increased
Obese I	30.0–34.9	Moderate
Obese II	35.0–39.9	Severe
Obese III	≥40.0	Very severe

Source: World Health Organization (2000).
BMI = body mass index.

Diabetes mellitus

The term 'diabetes mellitus' refers to a group of metabolic disorders, of which the two main types are insulin-dependent diabetes (type I) and non–insulin-dependent diabetes (type II) diabetes. Type I diabetes is brought about by a lack of insulin production and subsequent high plasma glucose (high blood sugar), known as hyperglycaemia. Type II diabetes occurs as a result of insufficient insulin or insulin resistance, meaning the body is unable to respond to the presence of insulin, reducing glucose uptake by muscle fibres and adipocytes.

Both obesity and body fat patterning are known risk factors for type II diabetes. Whilst not all overweight or obese individuals develop diabetes, a high proportion of type II diabetics are overweight or obese. Insulin resistance is one likely causal factor. Weight loss is often seen with type I diabetics, whereas weight gain is a common symptom of type II diabetes. Increased urination is common in both, as the body attempts to remove excess glucose. Common symptoms include increased thirst and hunger, and dehydration may occur. As a result, fluid shifts are often evident. Bone mineral density tends to be reduced in type I diabetics, but above-average in type II diabetics, likely due to high body mass. The reader is directed to the work of Stolarczyk & Heyward (2004) for an overview of the assessment of body composition in diabetic patients.

Thyroid dysfunction

Situated in the neck, the thyroid gland plays an important role in metabolism, as it produces the hormones that regulate metabolic rate. Problems occur when the gland is either underactive or overactive. The condition associated with an underactive thyroid gland is termed 'hypothyroidism', characterised by an under-production of thyroid hormones. The condition associated with an overactive thyroid gland is termed 'hyperthyroidism', in which there is an excess production of thyroid hormones.

In hypothyroidism, metabolic rate decreases and body weight tends to increase, often as a result of increased storage of body fat. Conversely, hyperthyroidism is associated with an increased metabolism and, unless energy intake meets the increased demand, body weight tends to decrease. In addition to fat loss, reductions may occur in muscle and bone mineral compartments. Fluid shifts may occur as a result of increased extracellular fluid.

Although relatively uncommon, it is also possible for individuals to suffer both forms of thyroid dysfunction, developing one form after the other, or fluctuating between phases of hypothyroid and hyperthyroid symptoms. The relationship between metabolic rate, energy balance and body composition is a complex one. It should be noted that different conclusions regarding the changes in body composition associated with thyroid disorders may be made depending on the method used to assess body composition (Lönn et al., 1998).

9.2.2 Cardiovascular and pulmonary diseases

Cardiovascular disease

Coronary heart disease, also known as coronary artery disease, is usually caused by a condition called 'atherosclerosis' in which fatty deposits on the walls of the arteries harden, forming plaques and restricting the flow of blood. Blood flow is reduced by arterial narrowing and plaques may break away, causing blockages in the circulatory system. These conditions may lead to angina, stroke or myocardial infarction (heart attack).

Obesity and abdominal adiposity are widely accepted as independent risk factors for cardiovascular disease, and many patients suffering cardiovascular disease are obese. Related risk factors include hypertension, insulin resistance and diabetes, abnormal blood lipid levels and physical inactivity. Once atherosclerosis has developed, individuals may further reduce physical activity due to symptoms such as chest pain and shortness of breath, often compounding the problem. Muscle mass may decrease through inactivity. In overweight individuals bone mineral density may be maintained due to skeletal loading.

Pulmonary disease

Pulmonary diseases may be restrictive, in which lung volume is reduced, or obstructive, in which airflow to the lungs is limited. One of the most common respiratory diseases is chronic obstructive pulmonary disease (COPD), which incorporates conditions such as emphysema and chronic bronchitis. Pulmonary diseases often bring about increased energy demand in breathing, but overall reduced physical activity, due to breathing difficulties. Peripheral muscle wasting and bone demineralisation commonly occur and the hydration of the fat-free mass may be reduced.

Cystic fibrosis (CF), whilst not solely a pulmonary disease, is an incurable condition characterised by frequent lung infections. Other systems, such as the digestive system, are also affected and an increased metabolic demand coupled with nutrient malabsorption means CF patients, the majority of whom are children, often fail to achieve 'normal' height and weight. Body fat and bone mineral density tend to be lower than in non-CF counterparts, and physical weakness is common. Further conditions may develop, such as CF-related diabetes and osteoporosis.

9.2.3 Wasting diseases

Wasting is defined as a state of non-volitional weight loss (Koch, 1998). The umbrella term 'wasting diseases' incorporates many disorders of different pathology, for example, neuromuscular diseases, cognitive/emotional disorders or immunological conditions. Whilst the various diseases differ in their aetiology, a brief overview is provided of some common issues affecting body composition.

Immunological/haematological disorders

Immunological/haematological disorders such as AIDS and cancer are often associated with changes in body mass and composition. The term 'cachexia' is used to describe the emaciation due to wasting and malnutrition often seen in patients with debilitating chronic disease. The specific 'HIV wasting syndrome' is defined as an involuntary loss of greater than 10 per cent baseline bodyweight, in addition to other HIV-related symptoms (Coodley, Loveless & Merrill, 1994). Loss of appetite, reduced energy intake and disorders such as metabolic dysfunction, problems with digestion and absorption, myopathy and other disease symptoms may contribute to weight loss. Whilst protein sparing may be observed during starvation in the absence of disease, HIV wasting is characterised by detrimental changes in the fat-free body compartment such as protein loss, leading to decreased muscle mass. Weight loss is common, particularly in patients who develop AIDS, and is associated with poorer clinical outcomes. In addition to changes brought about by disease, antiretroviral treatments are also associated with altered body composition. Changes in fat patterning are common in HIV patients, with some treatments associated with weight gain in the abdominal region, but wasting in the face and limbs. Fat deposits may also form at the base of the neck, resulting in a condition colloquially known as 'buffalo's hump'. Such redistribution of body fat stores is known as 'lipodystrophy'.

Cancer cachexia is characterised by loss of appetite, malabsorption of nutrients and weight loss, often with marked changes in body composition. Loss of appetite can occur as a cause, and partly a consequence, of malnourishment and metabolic abnormalities (Giacosa, Frascio, Sukkar & Roncella, 1996). Metabolic dysfunction includes alterations in the metabolism of protein, lipids and carbohydrates. As is the case with HIV-related wasting, cancer cachexia does not exhibit the protein-sparing that may be expected with decreased energy intake in the absence of physiological disease. Protein degradation takes place at a faster rate than that of protein synthesis and decreases are observed in skeletal muscle mass in addition to a loss of adipose tissue. Shifts in body water are evident, with an expansion of the extracellular mass. Cachexia affects nearly half of all cancer patients and is an important issue as it may impede responses to chemotherapy treatment and is associated with increased mortality (Esper & Harb, 2005).

9.2.4 Psychological disorders

The psychological disorder most commonly associated with body composition is anorexia nervosa, given its direct link with body image and severe restrictions in energy intake. It will be used as the example in this subsection, although many other psychological disorders can affect body composition, for example bulimia nervosa and binge-eating disorder. Other mental disorders and retardation may also impact upon body composition, for example, if an individual is incapable of feeding themselves properly.

It should be noted that the term 'anorexia', whilst colloquially used in reference to the disorder, is a clinical term meaning 'loss of appetite'; the term 'anorexia nervosa' refers specifically to the psychological eating disorder. Anorexia nervosa has a relatively high mortality rate compared to other eating disorders and psychiatric disorders in general. Arcelus, Mitchell, Wales & Nielsen (2011) evaluated data from 36 peer-reviewed studies, reporting an overall standardised mortality ratio (the ratio of observed to expected deaths) of 5.86, with one in five deaths in anorexic patients being attributed to suicide. Diagnostic criteria for anorexia nervosa include:

- Refusal to maintain 'normal' body weight; body weight falls below 85 per cent of expected weight for given age and height
- Intense fear of gaining weight, despite being underweight
- Distorted perception of body image; failure to recognise low body weight as problematic
- Amenorrhea (postmenarchal women).

(summarised from American Psychiatric Association, 2000)

Generally, metabolism slows in response to the reduction in energy intake and symptoms of malnutrition, such as hair loss and amenorrhoea in women, often occur. Preferential depletion of body fat stores is often evident in the early stages as the body attempts to preserve skeletal muscle through 'protein sparing'. However, subsequent weight loss also affects the fat-free compartment, for example, muscle mass and bone mineral mass decrease. Total body water may be reduced in absolute terms, but the proportion of body water to body mass may initially be greater, due to a primarily greater reduction in body fat than fat-free mass. The distributions of intra- and extra-cellular water may vary. Preferential depletion of subcutaneous fat may result in a greater visceral-to-total fat ratio.

9.2.5 Neuromuscular disease

Examples of neuromuscular disease include stroke, muscular dystrophy, multiple sclerosis and SCI; further details are provided in Section 9.3. Physical immobility causes muscular atrophy and increases in adiposity. The effect of neural impairment on the bone mineral compartment is termed 'neurogenic osteoporosis' and is evident in limbs no longer experiencing mechanical stimulation (gravitational loading and muscular contractions). Shifts may occur in tissue hydration, and total body water will tend to be lower than in healthy controls. Generally, the greater the physical impairment, the greater the impact on body composition.

9.3 Consequences of physical disability

9.3.1 Body composition in disability

Individuals with a physical disability, for example the wheelchair users pictured in Figure 9.1, offer a unique insight into the adaptive nature of human body composition. On a molecular level, disability results in changes to the proportions of total body protein, mineral and water, altering the density of the fat-free mass. Immobilisation and, in the case of paralysis, denervation result in muscular atrophy, reducing total body protein and the proportion of body mass composed of water. Inactivity and neural impairment lead to reduced bone mineral mass and, eventually, osteoporosis. In the case of SCI, such changes in body composition tend to occur below the level of injury, and are dependent upon the time, level and completeness of SCI. The basal metabolic rate is reduced, predominantly as a result of reductions in the fat-free mass. This and further reductions in energy expenditure resulting from immobility give a greater propensity for increased adiposity.

The changes in body composition associated with disability can be profound, and there is a clear need to be able to quantify and monitor changes accurately, particularly given the health risks associated with some conditions, for example

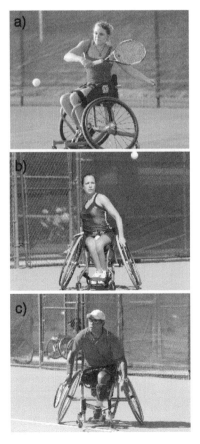

FIGURE 9.1 Wheelchair tennis players: (a) female with brittle bones; (b) female paraplegic; and (c) male with a single above-knee amputation (photographs courtesy of John Lenton).

there is an increased risk of coronary heart disease and type II diabetes in SCI patients. Not all changes in body composition associated with disability will be detrimental, for example everyday wheelchair use and engagement in physical activity and exercise programmes bring about muscular hypertrophy and help maintain/increase bone mineral density in the active regions of the body, despite atrophy and demineralisation continuing below the level of the lesion in SCI patients; this phenomenon can be seen in the case study presented in Section 9.3.3. Where possible, habitual physical activity is highly recommended, given its potential to improve body composition status and reduce the risks of adverse health consequences. For further information on exercise prescription in special populations, including SCI, the reader is referred to the work of Skinner (2005).

9.3.2 Paralympic classifications

From a sports perspective, the Paralympic Games developed from a rehabilitation programme for British Second World War veterans with SCI and, as evidenced by the 2008 Paralympics, the Games have progressed considerably. Now a stage for elite disabled athletes, the Paralympic Games include participants with a wide range of physical disabilities. For example, the team sport of wheelchair basketball is designed for athletes who have physical disabilities that prevent running, jumping and pivoting, such as paraplegia, amputations, or joint and musculo-skeletal conditions. (For a comprehensive introduction to the classification of wheelchair sport, the reader is referred to the work of Tweedy & Diaper, 2010.) Levels of participation in disability sport are also increasing at the recreational level.

Given the wide variety of disabilities seen amongst Paralympic athletes, there are several categories in which the athletes compete. The eligible disabilities for Paralympic competition are broken down into six broad categories. The categories are as follows:

- Amputee
- Cerebral palsy
- Intellectual disability
- Visual impairment
- Wheelchair
- Les Autres (a French term meaning 'others', who are athletes with disabilities that do not fall into the aforementioned categories; this category includes a range of conditions resulting in locomotive disorders, such as dwarfism or muscular dystrophy)

These categories are further broken down into classifications, which vary from sport to sport; the reader is referred to the International Paralympic Committee's classification manual for further information (IPC, 2007). For the purpose of conciseness, the focus in the present chapter is on three main groups: amputation, cerebral palsy and SCI.

A brief definition and the physiological and anatomical consequences of three main disability groups are shown in Table 9.2. These common disabilities can result from trauma or congenital birth complications, be caused by viral infections or toxic conditions, or arise from circulatory problems resulting in the loss of blood supply to a limb. Muscle atrophy in persons with either an amputation or SCI will be dependent upon not only the time of onset of the disability, but also the level of amputation and residual limb length, or level and completeness of the SCI, respectively. The American Spinal Injury Association (ASIA) use the dermatome chart, muscle function grading and impairment scale presented in Figure 9.2 to assess the level of neurological function in SCI individuals. Generic considerations and recommendations for the assessment of body composition of persons with these disabilities are highlighted in the final column of Table 9.2 and further detail is given in Section 9.4.

9.3.3 Body composition in SCI: a case study

The following case study demonstrates some differences in body shape and composition resulting from SCI. Differences in body composition between a female wheelchair athlete and an active, able-bodied woman of the same age and BMI are presented. Some of the SCI-associated changes in body composition actually affect body composition analysis and should be taken into account when interpreting results (see Section 9.4).

Quantitative results are shown in Table 9.3. Aside from the clear differences in posture shown in Figure 9.3, it can be seen that the wheelchair athlete has a higher proportion of fat-free soft tissue mass and corresponding lower proportion of fat mass, and greater bone mineral density in the upper limbs, as a result of activities of daily living and sport participation. Differences between individuals are even more notable in the lower body, with the wheelchair athlete demonstrating a higher relative fat mass, lower proportion of fat-free mass, and lower bone mineral density, consistent with the changes expected due to the muscle atrophy, bone demineralisation and increased fat storage associated with paralysis. Participation in physical activity does not prevent the adaptations to paralysis occurring below the level of injury. The results shown are typical of wheelchair athletes and must be taken into account when selecting an appropriate method of body composition analysis for use in this population. A whole-body approach (e.g. a measure of total percentage body fat) may produce 'normal' values, masking the marked differences between the upper and lower body, and techniques which use only part of the body (e.g. skinfold equations based on sites from just the upper body) may produce misleading results.

TABLE 9.2 Consequences of disability: amputation, cerebral palsy and SCI

Disability	Definition	Main exercise implications	Selected body composition considerations/tips
Amputation	Loss of limb(s) or portion of a limb(s) Examples: *Transtibial amputation* – below the knee *Transfemoral amputation* – above the knee	• Movement problems • Decreased gait efficiency • Problems with posture	• Errors associated with the measurement of height and weight due to the loss of limb(s) • Missing limbs may add error in meeting normative values assumed for pre-set equipment e.g. bioelectrical impedance and dual X-ray absorptiometry. Correction factors may be needed • Some individuals may be unable to hold the anatomical reference position for skinfolds e.g. upper body posture may be affected with development of shortened rhomboids • Depending upon the extent of the limb loss, postural imbalances may also be noted
Cerebral palsy	A non-progressive disorder caused by damage to the motor control areas of the brain which regulate neuromuscular function Example: *Hemiplegia* – paralysis on one side of the body	• Control of movement and posture can be affected • Abnormal muscle tone	• Increased muscular tone can often affect flexor and internal rotator muscles • Postural disorders develop in affected body segments that may prevent individuals holding the anatomical reference position • For scans during which movement must be avoided, problems may occur as some individuals may show continuous shaking and trembling

Disability	Definition	Main exercise implications	Selected body composition considerations/tips
Spinal cord injury	Complete or incomplete paralysis of the upper and/or lower extremities and the trunk resulting in impaired function. Examples: *Paraplegia* – lesion level of the spinal cord in or below the thoracic region. *Quadriplegia* – lesion level of the spinal cord in the cervical region. *Spina Bifida* – congenital spinal cord dysfunction (not caused through an acute injury to the spinal cord but through a lack of neural tube closure during development in the womb)	Muscle atrophy (decreased fat-free body mass). Changes in body fluid shifts due to loss of fat-free mass. Decreased functional capacity. Autonomic dysreflexia may occur in individuals with a SCI above lesion level T6. For the first two years following an SCI spasticity increases. This relates to an abnormal increase in muscle tone. Extended and poor wheelchair use/posture may result in contractures	Leg bags should be emptied prior to any measurement to avoid over-distending the bladder causing inaccuracies in the measurement of body mass. During transfers for any body composition assessment be aware of hypotension and dizziness and allow extra time to help with elevating the blood pressure. Avoid hard surfaces for extended periods of time (pressure sores). Curvature of the spine (scoliosis) may affect the accuracy of some of the skinfold measures of the sub-scapular region and left and right side comparisons. Some individuals may have problems with maintaining an appropriate posture and performing a maximal exhalation whilst fully submerged underwater. This is an important requirement for accurate measurement of body composition during hydrostatic weighing. The presence of surgical implants such as orthopaedic pins may affect the density of the fat-free mass. Some individuals may be unable to assume a supine position whilst on their back, affecting DXA and BIA. During DXA scans, some individual's natural posture may result in part of one leg overlapping the other. Radio-transparent foam padding should be inserted between the legs, so that the there is enough space for the placement of the segmental divisor lines during analysis.

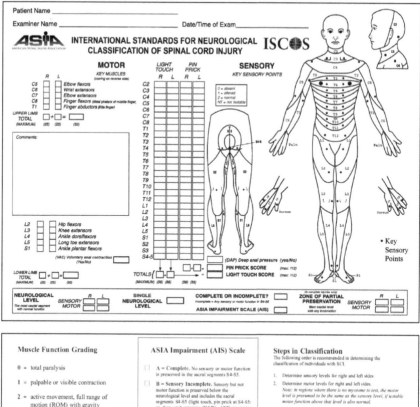

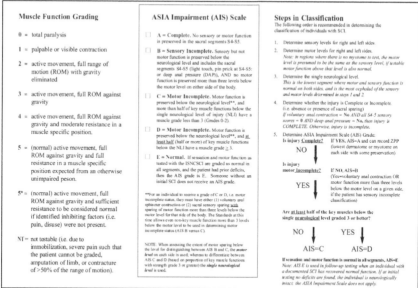

FIGURE 9.2 The American Spinal Injury Association *Standards for Neurological Classification of SCI* worksheet (source: American Spinal Injury Association: International Standards for Neurological Classification of Spinal Cord Injury, 2011; Atlanta, GA).

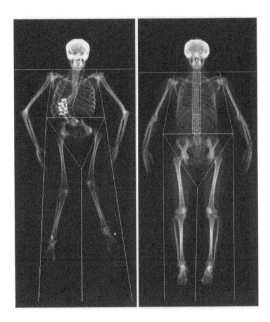

FIGURE 9.3 DXA scans of a female wheelchair athlete (L) and age- and BMI-matched able-bodied woman (R) (image © Laura Sutton).

TABLE 9.3 A comparison of DXA-determined body composition between a female wheelchair athlete and an age- and BMI-matched able-bodied reference woman

		Wheelchair athlete	*Reference woman*
Age (years)		33	33
Body mass index		19.6	20.0
FFST mass (%)	Arms	71.6	68.1
	Trunk	74.7	76.0
	Legs	47.4	69.4
	Total	67.1	72.5
Fat mass (%)	Arms	23.1	27.1
	Trunk	22.8	22.4
	Legs	49.4	26.8
	Total	28.6	24.0
BMD (g.cm^{-2})	Arms	0.927	0.719
	Trunk	–	0.821
	Legs	0.813	1.128
	Total	–	1.075

Notes

FFST = fat-free soft tissue.

BMD = bone mineral density.

Missing values reflect areas where orthopaedic implants preclude accurate determination of bone mineral content, area and areal density. (Metallic implants can be seen in Figure 9.3.)

9.4 General considerations for the assessment of body composition

The brief expositions in the present chapter should serve to highlight the fact that many diseases and disorders with adverse health consequences are associated with alterations to body composition, with changes occurring in various body compartments. In addition to variables such as age, gender, ethnicity, physical fitness etc. body composition status will vary in clinical populations according to the type, severity and duration of disease, further to any influence the treatment for the disease may exert upon the body. Unfortunately, there are currently no universally accepted guidelines as to how best to analyse and monitor changes in body composition for many clinical groups. In the remainder of the chapter, common methods of body composition analysis are considered in relation to their suitability for use with individuals with chronic disease/disability, with a particular focus on disabled athletes.

9.4.1 Densitometry

Densitometric methods, such as hydrodensitometry (hydrostatic, or underwater, weighing) and air displacement plethysmography (ADP, also known by the commercial name BodPod), are based on the classic two-compartment model of body composition. The two-compartment model relies on the assumption of relatively constant densities in the fat and fat-free mass. Assumptions are also made regarding the proportions of the different constituents comprising the fat-free mass, such as protein, mineral and water. The variability in these compartments discussed in Sections 9.2 and 9.3 means the validity of these approaches for the analysis of body composition may be compromised in many clinical groups. However, estimations of body density may be combined with other measures to provide multi-compartment models of body composition (see Section 9.4.3).

Hydrostatic weighing is not recommended for use in disability groups, as the procedure can be anxiety-producing and problems may be encountered when attempting to enter the tank, maintain an appropriate posture during assessment and perform a maximal exhalation whilst fully submerged underwater. Of the densitometric approaches, ADP may be more suitable; however, it has yet to be validated for use in disability groups and violations of assumptions, such as the assumed constant density of the fat-free mass, are common in such groups and may lead to inaccurate results. Densitometric methods tend not to be frequently used in the clinical setting, but techniques that have been calibrated against densitometric methods, such as bioelectric impedance analysis, may be employed, so the same considerations apply.

9.4.2 Dual X-ray absorptiometry

In addition to the provision of a three-compartment model of body composition, one of the main advantages of the use of DXA for body composition assessment in disease and disability groups is that it is not limited by the assumption of constant density of the fat-free mass, as is the traditional two-compartment densitometric model. Therefore, the method is more sensitive to the altered body composition often seen in these groups, such as bone demineralisation and changes in tissue hydration. Where conditions are associated with changes in the bone mineral compartment, DXA or medical imaging techniques such as computed tomography (CT) or magnetic resonance imaging (MRI) are recommended for use. However, even the accuracy of complex laboratory techniques may be reduced in certain conditions. For example, as discussed in Chapter 2.6, the phenomenon of 'beam hardening' which occurs as a result of tissue thickness reduces the accuracy of assessment by DXA in morbidly obese individuals.

Altered tissue hydration is relatively common in chronic disease, and it has been suggested that changes in the hydration of the fat-free mass could affect the accuracy of the estimation of body fat using DXA. Having considered both theoretical and empirical findings, Lohman, Harris, Teixeira & Weiss (2000) suggested that a change in water content of around 5 per cent could affect estimates of body fat by DXA by approximately 1–2.5 per cent. In general, the effect should not be so large as to preclude the use of DXA in clinical populations. The presence of surgical implants such as orthopaedic pins will attenuate X-ray beams and produce spurious results. However, whilst such artefacts often cannot be removed, they are usually visible during the analysis stages of a DXA assessment and, therefore, adjustments can be undertaken during analysis to account for their presence. The DXA method has been validated for use SCI and many chronic diseases.

Other issues to consider include whether or not the participant can assume the standard scan position. It is important to replicate the position as closely as possible, but without causing undue discomfort to the participant. If malformation or disability prevents a participant from assuming the standard position, radiotransparent materials may be used to aid positioning. Suitable materials may be identified by simply performing a scan with just the material in the scan field to ensure the software reports zero values for all compartments. Some conditions will cause the participant to experience spasms or extreme discomfort, which may prevent them from maintaining a still, supine position for the scan duration. During the analysis stages, care should be taken when placing segmental divisor lines. If these cannot be placed optimally, care should be taken when interpreting segmental values, for example, comparing left and right limbs, as the demarcation may not be identical in each case.

It is worth noting that CT and magnetic resonance techniques can provide a more detailed analysis than DXA, but these complex methods are still not free from underlying assumptions. The instruments quantify areas and volumes and therefore require an assumed tissue density in order to convert them into mass. Results will also be affected by the presence of artefacts. These complex methods are frequently used in the clinical context, but are generally not readily available in other settings, so tend not to be considered common methods of body composition assessment.

9.4.3 Multi-compartment models

Multi-compartment modelling is widely considered to provide the current 'gold standard' approach to body composition analysis in healthy population groups. Various multi-compartment models have been proposed, with different numbers of compartments and definitions of the compartmental breakdown. The most common approach is a four-compartment model dividing the body into protein, mineral, water and fat. Techniques are combined to produce the different measurements, for example mineral mass may be estimated using DXA and total body water may be estimated via isotopic dilution. Protein and fat mass may be differentiated using measurements of body density; alternatively, techniques such as *in vivo* neutron activation analysis may be used to estimate protein mass directly, allowing body fat to be determined by subtracting the fat-free mass estimates from the total body weight. Equations are employed to estimate the necessary compartments and provide the final body composition model.

The more compartments accounted for in the model, the greater the possibility of accounting for deviations from assumed proportions and densities compared to models with fewer components, and the greater the sensitivity to changes in body composition. Therefore, for patients with conditions known to elicit changes in the fat-free mass, such as changes to tissue hydration and reductions in bone mineral content or protein mass, multi-compartment models are highly recommended. However, a 'trade-off' occurs, as the more complex the model, the more advanced the technology required and the greater the cost, both in time and finance, rendering the multi-compartment approach unrealistic in many settings. Moreover, more advanced techniques such as whole-body counting and *in vivo* neutron activation analysis tend to be harder to come by.

9.4.4 Bioelectric impedance analysis

Bioelectrical impedance is based on the principle that fat mass, containing very little water, impedes an electric signal, whereas fat-free mass, with a high water content of approximately 73 per cent (Wang et al., 1999) conducts the signal. The impedance value is combined with values for height, mass and estimated frame size to calculate body water content and compute fat and fat-free mass. Assumptions are that the water content of both fat and fat-free mass is constant, and that hydration levels do not differ significantly between individuals, an assumption which may be violated in disabled populations and other clinical groups. Furthermore, significant differences in impedance values are brought about when measurements are taken with the participant in a seated position as opposed to a supine posture. This could pose problems, for example, for wheelchair users unable to adopt the standard supine measurement position (Allison, Singer & Marshall, 1995). Furthermore, it may be difficult to obtain an accurate measure of height in individuals with postural abnormalities.

Often, equations are validated for use with specific conditions, for example, anorexia nervosa. When working with clinical patients in settings where so-called 'gold standard' techniques are not available, it is recommended that it be checked whether field-based equations have been validated and, if so, that the reference method used will not have been compromised by the anatomical/physiological consequences of the condition. Bioelectric impedance analysis is sometimes used in clinical settings to assess total-body water or its constituent intra- and extra-cellular compartments. From estimations of water compartments, body cell mass can be predicted. Measurements of total-body resistance and reactance are used to compute a 'phase angle' measurement, which may be used to assess overall health and monitor disease.

9.4.5 Anthropometry

Due to differences in body composition and fat patterning, conventional skinfold equations may not be applicable in disabled and diseased populations. Often, skinfold equations are only valid in the population from which they were derived, so equations developed using 'healthy' members of the general population will lack transferability to chronic disease patients. For example, generalised equations have been shown to overestimate body density and underestimate relative fat in disability groups (Maggioni et al., 2003).

In conditions associated with altered fat patterning, such as HIV lipodystrophy, it is recommended that generalised anthropometric equations not be used for the prediction of percentage body fat. Equations rely on certain sites and assumptions of a relationship between those sites and total body fat. Given the deviations from 'standard' fat patterning associated with some clinical conditions, such prediction equations may lack accuracy and sensitivity to change in body composition.

In the absence of specific, validated equations, anthropometric measurements without subsequent conversion to percentage body fat estimates may prove adequate for the assessment of changes in body composition in disabled individuals. Examples of such measurements include measurements of weight, skinfold thickness and circumferences. Monitoring of body weight or BMI alone is rarely sufficient, but if weight were to change, inspection of changes to skinfold and circumference measurements should provide an indication of whether the change has occurred in the fat or fat-free compartment. However, this is a crude approach, and may lack sensitivity to certain changes, such as changes in tissue hydration.

It is important that longitudinal measurements be carried out with as much consistency as possible to allow for the accurate and reliable monitoring of changes in body composition. Some conditions will actually preclude the use of the technique, for example, skinfold calliper jaws may not open wide enough to take valid skinfold measurements in morbidly obese individuals.

Circumference measurements such as waist girth and the waist-to-hip ratio are often used to predict cardiovascular disease risk in able-bodied individuals. However, due to muscle paralysis and atrophy, circumference measurements may lack predictive ability in disability groups. As such, it is recommended that they are predominantly used for the monitoring of changes in body shape and size until they have been validated for use in disease risk prediction.

9.4.6 Body mass index

It is well-established that the body mass index (BMI) is limited by its inability to reflect body composition, a limitation which is relevant in many clinical groups. The measure is correlated with conditions such as obesity, diabetes and cardiovascular risk factors, so may be useful as a screening tool, given that it is inexpensive, and quick and easy to use. For these reasons, it is often used in clinical settings, and has been deemed sufficiently sensitive in certain groups, for example the identification of over-fat children (Daniels, 2009). However, BMI will lack sensitivity in groups in which increases in adiposity are coupled with decreases in fat-free body mass, or whose body shape and size is markedly different from normative or expected values.

Unsurprisingly, it has been shown that anthropometric measures such as BMI are poor predictors of body fat in children with moderate to severe cerebral palsy (Kuperminc et al., 2010). However, this is a group of individuals whom clinical dietitians may monitor carefully, as many children with cerebral palsy have been reported as underweight, given the increased metabolic demands from spastic muscles and energy expenditure in performing daily tasks.

Tzamaloukas, Patron & Malhotra (1994) provided an overview of how amputation may affect the calculation of BMI if corrections are not made. This uncorrected BMI is computed in amputees as actual (post-amputation) weight divided by the square of actual (post-amputation) height. The authors provided an overview of three situations, which include one in which amputation does not affect height and two in which height is affected by amputation of the legs, either at the same or different lengths. It appears that the success of using BMI is heavily reliant upon correcting the BMI equation based on the fraction of body weight lost to amputation. The reader is referred to the publication of Tzamaloukas et al. for further information regarding equations that allow for corrections for limb loss.

Body mass index is generally not considered a valid indicator of body fat levels in paraplegic individuals. Body fat tends to be underestimated, and Buchholz, McGillivray & Pencharz (2003) found that the BMI cut-off value of $30\,kg.m^{-2}$ (obese category) correctly identified only 20 per cent of obese paraplegic subjects. The relative content and density of the different body compartments is highly variable in disability groups. Further measurement error may be introduced when trying to obtain height and weight measurements in individuals with limited mobility and altered posture. For a review of further work with sedentary and recreationally active SCI groups, the reader is directed to the review article of Buchholz & Bugaresti (2005). Further research is warranted to identify new BMI categories for persons with an SCI.

Conclusion

The ability to quantify and monitor changes in body composition is important in clinical populations. However, chronic disease and disability result in anatomical and physiological adaptations that can make the selection of an appropriate, valid method of analysis difficult. In many cases, the equipment and finances available may limit the choice of assessment techniques, although the best efforts should be made to find methods that have been sufficiently validated for the population of interest. The body compartment of interest may also help guide the choice of assessment technique.

Of the current, more commonly used approaches, DXA is preferred over methods relying on the two-compartment model, but cannot be considered a 'gold standard' approach at present. Despite the greater inconvenience in obtaining measurements, more complex laboratory techniques and multi-compartment models provide the most promising methods of body composition analysis for diseased and disabled individuals and are recommended for use, where possible. Such approaches should also prove useful in the provision of reference methods for the calibration and validation of less complex and/or more portable instruments for subsequent use in clinical population groups.

References

Allison, G.T., Singer, K.P. and Marshall, R.N. (1995). The effect of body position on bioelectrical resistance in individuals with spinal cord injury. *Disability and Rehabilitation, 17*, 424–429.

American Psychiatric Association. (2000). *DSM-IV-TR: Diagnostic and Statistical Manual of Mental Disorders (Text Revision)*. Washington, DC: American Psychiatric Publishing, Inc.

Arcelus, J., Mitchell, A.J., Wales, J. and Nielsen, S. (2011). Mortality rates in patients with anorexia nervosa and other eating disorders. *Archives of General Psychiatry, 68*, 724–731.

Buchholz, A.C. and Bugaresti, J.M. (2005). A review of body mass index and waist circumference as markers of obesity and coronary heart disease risk in persons with chronic spinal cord injury. *Spinal Cord, 43*, 513–518.

Buchholz, A.C., McGillivray, C.F. and Pencharz, P.B. (2003). The use of bioelectric impedance analysis to measure fluid compartments in subjects with chronic paraplegia. *Archives of Physical Medicine and Rehabilitation, 84*, 854–861.

Coodley, G.O., Loveless, M.O. and Merrill, T.M. (1994). The HIV wasting syndrome: a review. *Journal of Acquired Immune Deficiency Syndromes, 7*, 681–694.

Daniels, S.R. (2009). The use of BMI in the clinical setting. *Pediatrics, 124*, S35–S41.

Esper, D.H. and Harb, W.A. (2005). The cancer cachexia syndrome: a review of metabolic and clinical manifestations. *Nutrition in Clinical Practice, 20*, 369–376.

Giacosa, A., Frascio, F., Sukkar, S.G. and Roncella, S. (1996). Food intake and body composition in cancer cachexia. *Nutrition, 12*, S20–S23.

IPC (International Paralympic Committee). (2007). *IPC Classification Code and International Standards*. Bonn: IPC.

Kissebah, A.H. and Krakower, G.R. (1994). Regional adiposity and morbidity. *Physiological Reviews, 74*, 761–811.

Koch, J. (1998). The role of body composition measurements in wasting syndromes. *Seminars in Oncology, 25*, S12–S19.

Kuperminc, M.N., Gurka, M.J., Bennis, J.A., Busby, M.G., Grossberg, R., Henderson, R.C. et al. (2010). Anthropometric measures: poor predictors of body fat in children with moderate to severe cerebral palsy. *Development Medicine and Child Neurology, 52*, 824–830.

Lohman, T.G., Harris, M., Teixeira, P.J. and Weiss, L. (2000). Assessing body composition and changes in body composition. Another look at dual-energy X-ray absorptiometry. *Annals of the New York Academy of Sciences, 904*, 45–54.

Lönn, L., Stenlöf, K., Ottosson, M., Lindroos, A., Nyström, E. and Sjöström, L. (1998). Body weight and body composition changes after treatment of hyperthyroidism. *The Journal of Clinical Endocrinology and Metabolism, 83*, 4269–4273.

Maggioni, M., Bertoli, S., Margonato, V., Merati, G., Veicsteinas, A. and Testolin, G. (2003). Body composition assessment in spinal cord injury subjects. *Acta Diabetologica, 40*, S183–S186.

Schutte, J.E., Townsend, E.J., Hugg, J., Shoup, R.F., Malina, R.M. and Blomqvist, C.G. (1984). *Journal of Applied Physiology, 56*, 1647–1649.

Skinner, J.S. (2005). *Exercise Testing and Exercise Prescription for Special Cases: Theoretical Basis and Clinical Application* (Revised 3rd edition). Philadelphia, PA: Lippincott, Williams & Wilkins.

Stolarczyk, L.M. and Heyward, V.H. (2004). Assessing body composition of adults with diabetes. *Diabetes Technology and Therapeutics, 1*, 289–296.

Tweedy, S. and Diaper, N. (2010). Introduction to wheelchair sport. In V. Goosey-Tolfrey (Ed.) *Wheelchair Sport* (pp. 3–28). Champaign, IL: Human Kinetics.

Tzamaloukas, A.H., Patron, A. and Malhotra, D. (1994). Body mass index in amputees. *Journal of Parenteral and Enteral Nutrition, 18*, 355–358.

Wang, Z., Deurenberg, P., Wang, W., Pietrobelli, A., Baumgartner, R.N. and Heymsfield, S.B. (1999). Hydration of fat-free body mass: review and critique of a classic body-composition constant. *American Journal of Clinical Nutrition, 69*, 833–841.

WHO (World Health Organization). (2000). Obesity: preventing and managing the global epidemic. *Report of a WHO Consultation. WHO Technical Report Series 894.* Geneva: WHO.

10

BODY COMPOSITION
Professional practice and
an interdisciplinary toolkit

Laura Sutton and Arthur D. Stewart

This chapter will cover:

10.1 Professional standards

What do we mean by professional? Using the commonly understood meaning, skilled or competent, or main income-generating occupation, it is hard to envisage what a body composition professional is. However, if we consider a research scientist, clinical dietitian, sports coach or human biologist, we immediately recognise that such a profession has associated expectations. There are expectations of conduct, in the way individuals are treated; there are expectations of being capable of executing specified tasks, and expectations concerning how both individuals and tasks are managed. Part of the richness of body composition lies in the diversity of its origins and, although professionalism spans each of its disciplines, there are common principles, but also distinct differences in expectation between the different professions which use body composition measures.

Common principles would embrace traits such as honesty, trustworthiness and a recognition of the governance frameworks of the profession. A research scientist would not be able to carry out data collection for a study without ethical permission from the academic institution or the local health authority. However, the sports coach, whose body composition measures are being made on athletes as a matter of monitoring of training programmes could argue that such permission is not strictly necessary. Without doubt, individuals have a right to be protected from unscrupulous research where they are subjected to prolonged, uncomfortable or even dangerous procedures, and as a consequence we have seen a dramatic tightening of legislative and governance arrangements in most countries over the last two decades. Many researchers are daunted at the prospect of submitting their first health authority ethics application, due to the complexity of the process and the wide consideration necessary to understand the implications of the research. However, such a process exists to protect both the research volunteer and the researcher, by enabling difficulties to be foreseen and appropriate action to be taken.

Common principles also extend to competent literacy, numeracy, record keeping and audit of not only of data acquisition, but of the process of staff training and the qualifications record of employees. Increasingly, competence requires a demonstrable evidence base for dealing with untoward situations, where individuals participating may complain, or be harmed physically or psychologically. Standards relating to health and safety, ethics and good practice are explored further in Section 10.3.

10.2 A bridge-builder between disciplines

The analysis of body composition takes places across a vast number of different, but often interlinking, fields, including, but not limited to: medicine, anthropology, nutrition, ergonomics, biomechanics and exercise physiology. One of the most exciting aspects of being involved in academic research is the interplay between different specialisations, and body composition specialists can often find themselves working across a variety of settings.

As interdisciplinary collaborations have proved essential in understanding the range of increasingly complex challenges facing science and medicine today, techniques are developed that are essentially enabling technologies, which assist solving problems in one discipline, using techniques from another. Indeed, many of the techniques implemented today in sport, exercise and health settings have been 'borrowed' from other disciplines, and sometimes developed further. For example, attempts to standardise manual anthropometric measurements were initially made in the nineteenth century in order to identify individuals for policing and crime-fighting, prior to the development of more modern techniques such as fingerprinting and DNA analysis. Other anthropometric techniques were developed and used, somewhat controversially, by eugenicists in the twentieth century, looking to determine physical differences and superiority/inferiority between races. Now commonly used to assess body shape, size and composition in sport, exercise and health settings across the globe, anthropometric methods have been developed and standardised to a very high level.

The first widespread use of whole-body counting was in nuclear power plants, to monitor the radiation exposure of the workers. The ability to quantify different chemicals in the human body to a high degree of accuracy made gamma-counting techniques, such as whole-body counting and *in vivo* neutron activation analysis, ideal candidates for reference methods of body composition analysis, and they have since proven invaluable in the validation of newer, less complex methods. Other interesting crossovers between disciplines include the use of similar body scanning techniques in obesity clinics and research laboratories as may be found in the clothing manufacturing industry.

Now routinely considered one of the reference methods of body composition analysis, dual X-ray absorptiometry (DXA) was originally developed as a bone densitometry technique for clinical settings. Indeed, DXA still provides the gold standard method for the diagnosis and monitoring of osteoporosis. However, given its ability to determine the relative proportions of fat and fat-free soft tissue mass in addition to differentiating bone mineral from non-bone material, DXA has become a useful technique for three-compartmental body composition analysis. Another technique borrowed from medical settings and sometimes used in body composition analysis is ultrasonography. Predominantly used in medicine for diagnostic or therapeutic purposes, ultrasound instruments may also be used to estimate percentage body fat in a manner similar to the caliper method, and the development of portable devices makes ultrasound a promising field-based method for the two-compartmental analysis of body composition.

Thus, it can be seen that body composition analysis, and the various measurement tools involved, play an important role in many distinct settings. Body composition analysis remains a dynamic field, as new applications are constantly being developed. It is now possible to quantify all of the major body components *in vivo*, whether it be on a chemical or anatomical level, so we look to the future for the introduction of new technologies, the improvement of existing tools, and the continuation of interdisciplinary links and discovery of new uses for methods of body composition analysis.

10.3 Health, safety and ethical considerations

10.3.1 Training

In order to ensure optimal safety and good practice, it is essential that a practitioner has good knowledge of the procedures to be followed, and demonstrates competency and confidence in their execution. An assessor who demonstrates these traits is more likely to put a participant at ease, which should aid compliance and help achieve high quality measurements, giving more valid and reliable results.

Not all methods of body composition assessment carry specific training requirements, so it is often left to the individual or organisation to define the amount of practice and learning required before an operator may be deemed competent and capable of carrying out assessments on others. Examples of methods with no specific or legal training requirements include commercially available measurement tools such as bioelectric impedance analysis (BIA) and anthropometry kits. Where no formal training programmes exist, it is advisable that the user reads fully any information manual or provided literature, and practises sufficiently to ensure proficiency and to minimise operator measurement error when using the equipment with clients.

In the case of anthropometry, bespoke accreditation schemes are available (see Section 10.5) and it is highly advisable that training be sought. If techniques such as the correct manipulation of skinfold calipers have not been demonstrated and practised, there is a greater risk of discomfort for the participant, in addition to a higher error of measurement, reducing the validity of the results. An example of causing harm to the participant from improper use of equipment is if the skinfold caliper and the skinfold site were not held correctly, as if the grip is lost and the skin pinched by the calipers, the participant is highly likely to feel discomfort. For anthropometrists who have not undergone formal training, it is still advised that ISAK procedures be followed, and practice be carried out in a bid to reduce the technical error of measurement.

There is no widely recognised accreditation scheme for hydrodensitometry (hydrostatic or underwater weighing), and most centres will provide in-house training. It is not unusual for participants to feel some vulnerability during hydrodensitometry, particularly if it is their first time, given the requirement of full submersion and maximal exhalation underwater. Thus, it is essential that the assessor be able to explain the procedure fully, demonstrate techniques where necessary, and ensure the participant is willing and able to comply. Practice and experience enable the assessor to determine when a measurement is suboptimal and make it possible for him/her to coach the participant, increasing the validity and reliability of the results obtained.

When conducting hydrodensitometric assessments, it is a health and safety requirement that a third person be present, so that in the event of a participant becoming uncomfortable or distressed, one person is able to remain with the participant whilst the other seeks help, if necessary. Other aspects of preparing the apparatus for measurement require careful attention, such as cleaning and sterilisation, electrical isolation of the tank heater, mixing pump and load cell, and the practicalities of minimising the spread of water from the participant emerging from the tank after the measurement.

An example of a common method of assessment that does require formal training prior to use is DXA. It is common for DXA operators to undergo two forms of training: training with the instrument, often provided by the manufacturer, and radiation training, to ensure the operator is aware of the risks and the regulations which must be followed. Regulation 11 of the Ionising Radiation (Medical Exposure) Regulations (Department of Health, 2000) prohibits any practitioner from carrying out procedures without having undertaken adequate training. Adherence to local radiologic safety requirements is essential, so it is recommended that a local radiation protection officer be contacted to provide the required information and training. Locally-written protocols are a legal requirement, and quality control procedures should also be developed and adhered to (Ryan, 2003). Operators should be able to provide evidence of training, if required, and records of work carried out, for auditing purposes. It is important that operators have good knowledge of the technique and are able to interpret output; however, if an operator is not medically trained, s/he may not make diagnoses, but should refer the participant to an appropriate clinician, should s/he detect any anomalies in test results.

The International Society for Clinical Densitometry (ISCD, 2007) recommends that technologists perform precision assessments after learning basic scanning skills, and advises that operators retrain if the precision error is too great. (That which constitutes an unacceptable margin of error should be predetermined, and may differ depending on the centre and the purpose of the assessment.) Indeed, ensuring low intra- and inter-operator error should be considered standard practice, irrespective of the method of assessment. In all areas, knowledge and competence should be kept up-to-date with appropriate continued professional development and training, and membership of professionally recognised bodies, where appropriate.

10.3.2 Assessing risk

A risk assessment is an evaluation of the potential causes of harm, conducted in a bid to protect people. It is often a legal requirement, particularly in the workplace. The Health and Safety Executive (HSE; the British independent watchdog for work-related health) identifies the following five steps to conducting a risk assessment:

1. Identify the hazards
2. Decide who might be harmed and how
3. Evaluate the risks and decide on precaution
4. Record your findings and implement them
5. Review your assessment and update if necessary

(HSE, 2011)

An example of a basic risk assessment form, acceptable in a university setting, is provided in Appendix 10.4. A hazard is defined as that which may cause harm, and risk takes into account the chance and severity of harm from the hazard.

Whilst a risk assessment form might suffice for some methods of body composition assessment, others often require further health and safety consider-ations, for example radiographic methods. In the UK, given that radiation is a hazardous substance, the completion of a COSHH form (Control of Substances Hazardous to Health) may be required in addition to a generic risk assessment form. Further information on COSHH can be obtained from the HSE website (www.hse.gov.uk). Other safety measures must also be followed, for example operators should wear radiation dosimeter badges, to be checked regularly to ensure 'safe' exposure levels, and dosimeters should also be placed in close proximity to the instrument to check for radiation leaks. A radiation 'trefoil' sign should be placed on the door, which should remain closed during assessments. Instruments should be serviced, typically bi-annually, to ensure safe operation. Radiation scatter can be checked during routine servicing. Service logs should be maintained and quality control procedures, such as system calibrations, should be carried out in accordance with manufacturer guidelines. A radiation protection advisor must approve a site for scanning to occur and a local radiation protection supervisor should ensure compliance with local radiation safety rules (Ryan, 2003).

10.3.3 Ethics

Ethics can be considered a system of moral principles. Most centres, such as hospitals and universities, will have an institutional ethics committee or review board, tasked with ensuring the safety and well-being of patients or participants taking part in research. In the UK, there is also a National Research Ethics Service (NRES), which aims to facilitate and promote ethical research.

Many now infamous cases highlight the need for the ethical control of research. Such cases include experimentation at Unit 731 in Japan (1935–1945), the Nazi research programme during the Second World War and the Tuskegee Syphilis Experiment carried out in the USA (1932–1972), amongst others. The Nuremberg Trials which took place after the Second World War led to the development of the Nuremberg Code, which outlined ethical principles for human experimentation. Important conditions included the need for voluntary informed consent from participants and a valid research design, capable of producing results to the benefit of society (NIH, 2004). The World Medical Association subsequently published a statement of ethical principles for medical research, based on the Nuremberg Code, known as the Declaration of Helsinki. Another important publication was the Belmont Report, a set of guidelines for human experimentation, published in the USA in 1979. Three fundamental principles identified in the Belmont Report are:

- Respect for persons
- Beneficence
- Justice

(National Commission for the Protection of Human Subjects of Biomedical and Behavioral Research, 1979)

Therefore, participants should be informed of what to expect and it should be confirmed that they have understood the explanation prior to providing voluntary consent. An example voluntary consent form is presented in Appendix 10.3. The form provided is fairly rigorous and simpler forms may be appropriate in some circumstances, for example within universities using healthy adult volunteers.

Participants should be protected, treated fairly and not exploited in any way. Benefits to participants should be maximised, whilst the risk of harm should be minimised. There may be extra safeguards necessary where the participants are in a dependent relationship with the researcher, for instance with university undergraduate students volunteering for research undertaken by a tutor.

Most local ethical guidelines were developed in line with the principles outlined in the aforementioned historic documents. Ethics panels now exist to ensure ethical principles are adhered to, focusing on participants' rights, dignity, safety and welfare. Research proposals are checked to ensure they comply with local and national codes of practice, and participant recruitment must not be initiated until approval has been granted. When completing a risk assessment and making an application to an ethics committee, it is essential to include information of any 'special populations' (see Section 10.4) who may be involved, accounting for any specific requirements. In the UK, approval should be sought from a local research ethics committee (LREC) and, if the research is to involve NHS patients, staff or facilities, NRES approval is also required. Ethical approval may also be required in other instances, for example for the use of invasive practices when teaching or training others, and even when approval is not required, it can be helpful to have confirmation of this.

Any data collected and stored must be in accordance with the necessary legislation. In the UK, the processing of data relating to individuals must be conducted in accordance with the Data Protection Act of 1998. Individual centres may also have local data protection policies. In general, personal data should be anonymised where possible, with information stored according to a participant code to ensure data cannot be related back to a particular individual. Data must be kept confidential and stored in a secure location, allowing for retrieval and, if necessary, demonstration of the validity of the data. Some centres will specify a time period for which primary data must be stored prior to deletion, for example a period of five years. Personal data must not be kept any longer than necessary. It should be decided prior to data collection how the information will be stored and who will be permitted access to the data. Electronic data should be regularly backed up, with replicate data sets stored in a different location to the original data to ensure minimal loss in the event of damage. Encryption may be required for backing up sensitive data. Research databases may be submitted for ethical review on a voluntary basis, as approval is only required by legislation if identifiable data are being processed without consent.

10.3.4 Other aspects of good practice

Even once approval for conducting certain procedures has been granted following ethical review, ethical considerations must continually be made in the workplace. Explicit ethical requirements include, for example, obtaining informed consent from participants, conducting risk assessments to protect them from harm and ensuring the secure storage of data. However, there are other, more implicit, rules of conduct when working with clients. A certain etiquette must be observed in order to put clients at ease and observe any personal boundaries.

The term 'proxemics' refers to personal space issues and relates to other aspects of behaviour and non-verbal communication that may be considered when interacting with a client, such as posture, eye contact, volume of speech and physical proximity. 'Haptics' refers to touching behaviours which is usually an inevitable component of measuring. Both proxemics and haptics are interpreted differently under different cultures, and it is important to be sensitive to this. It is often helpful for the assessor to inform the client what s/he is about to do immediately prior to doing it, and have the client respond, and indicate if, at any stage, s/he begins to feel uncomfortable.

Such ethnic and cultural sensitivities considerations are of particular importance in body composition assessment, which often requires the client to wear minimal clothing and may involve palpation, marking and grasping of surface tissues. In certain cultures, codes of dress may apply, and it may be inappropriate for individuals of opposite gender to come into close proximity or contact.

Privacy must be respected at all times and personal information must not be divulged unless permission has been granted by the individual. It is essential that the assessor, or individual tasked with relaying the results of a body composition assessment, demonstrate sensitivity and tact when feeding back information, as body issues are often a personal and sometimes embarrassing concern for some. Sensitivity is of particular importance when dealing with emotionally vulnerable clients, for example sufferers of eating disorders, as comments may trigger or reinforce undesirable behaviour.

10.4 Working with special populations

There is no universal definition of what constitutes a so-called 'special' population, but in sport, exercise and health settings, special populations are often taken to be groups of individuals with distinct features that distinguish them from characteristics of the 'general' population. Typically defined, special groups often account for a large proportion of the population, and may include women (particularly pregnant or breastfeeding women), children, the elderly and individuals with injuries or chronic disease. Such groups may be more sensitive or vulnerable, and specific considerations may need to be made when conducting body composition assessments.

When working with special populations, it is important to endeavour to identify beforehand any special requirements, issues with particular measurement techniques and amendments that may need to be made to normal assessment procedures. For example, it is important to ensure women are not pregnant or breastfeeding prior to exposing them to ionising radiation, or to enquire as to whether an individual has a pacemaker prior to using bioelectric impedance analysis. Often certain groups have a tendency to violate the underlying assumptions of a particular method, which may preclude its use, for example bone demineralisation in elderly or paralysed individuals means constancy of the fat-free mass cannot be assumed, so two-compartment techniques such as hydrostatic weighing may not be advisable. The reader is referred to Chapter 9 for examples of common considerations that need to be made when working with chronic disease and disability groups. In many cases, it may just be that certain individuals are less mobile and require more time and assistance when undergoing assessment. An example of the assessment of body composition in a special population group is shown in Figure 10.1. In this example, the standard measurement position for the iliac crest skinfold recommended by the International Society for the Advancement of Kinanthropometry (ISAK) has been adapted to allow the measurement to be taken from a spinal cord-injured individual.

A child is commonly defined as an individual under the age of 16 (e.g. Scotland) or 18 (e.g. England and Wales). When working with children in the UK, it is essential to obtain a disclosure form from the Criminal Records Bureau. In other

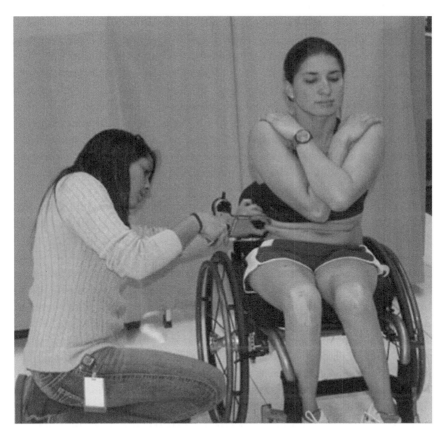

FIGURE 10.1 In athletes with lower spinal cord injuries which preclude ISAK's upright posture, it is possible to standardise measurements by having the individual sitting up straight, without support (photograph © Alicia Kendig, United States Olympic Committee).

countries, national requirements should be checked prior to the arrangement of assessment sessions. The informed consent of a parent or guardian should also be obtained prior to assessment. Many individuals, whilst still classified as children, are capable of understanding and voluntarily consenting to procedures, however, information should still be relayed to the individual(s) in the parental role. When explaining procedures to younger children, it is essential to use terminology they can understand. In laboratory settings it is not uncommon for children to feel intimidated by the surroundings, so it is important to engage with them in an attempt to put them at ease. When interpreting the results of a body composition assessment, it is imperative not to employ normative values or reference ranges based on adult populations, but to provide norms and recommendations based on age or the level of growth or maturation, where possible. It should be borne in mind that the use of some methods of assessment may prove more difficult with children compared to adults, for example methods in which the participant is required to remain still for a certain length of time.

For adults who are mentally incapable of providing voluntary informed consent to undergo body composition analysis, informed consent may be obtained from the person given the rights to the individual's health care. This person is most likely to be a relative, but in some cases may be the manager of a care home or a court-appointed receiver. When working with individuals with cognitive or intellectual disability, it is advisable to research the condition in order to determine how best to interact with the individual, and understand any behavioural issues s/he may have. What may seem completely routine for a healthy adult might invoke a stress response in those with cognitive impairment and assessments should be closely monitored and interrupted if the participant appears to show signs of undue distress.

It could be argued that women do not form a special population, given that women account for approximately half the general population. However, from an assessment perspective, additional considerations do need to be made when working with women, compared to their male counterparts, in light of the potentially intrusive questioning some approaches necessarily involve. Screening questionnaires are recommended to determine whether a woman is pregnant or breastfeeding, and it should be checked whether the planned method of assessment is appropriate in such cases. In the case of DXA whole-body scanning, women should be asked to wear a bra without underwiring, or to remove their bra for the scan, as metal or plastic features often affect the scan and, due to the density of the material, the bone mineral content and density for the torso area are overestimated. Breast implants can also affect the quality of measurement as, for example, depending on the density, estimates of body fat by densitometric methods will differ, and silicone implants are incorrectly reported as bone mineral mass in DXA scanning (Madsen, Lorentzen, Lauridsen, Egsmose & Sorensen, 2000). Circamensal rhythms in postmenarchal, premenopausal women may affect some measures, given the differences in hydration status and body weight across the cycle, although in most cases such variation should prove negligible. It may be necessary to look for signs of the female athlete triad when working with female athletes. It should also be considered that most female participants may feel more comfortable working with a female practitioner, or having another woman present when undergoing assessment by a male practitioner.

10.5 Best practice example: ISAK

Founded in 1986, the International Society for the Advancement of Kinanthropometry (ISAK) is an organisation of individuals whose scientific and professional work is related to kinanthropometry. The Society succeeded the International Working Group on Kinanthropometry, which was founded in 1978. It exists to develop and maintain a network of professionals measuring to a common protocol. In order to promote standardised anthropometric techniques and applications, ISAK runs an international accreditation scheme, used worldwide to train and accredit people in anthropometry. Information in this section is reproduced with permission from the ISAK Accreditation Scheme Handbook (Marfell-Jones, Olds, Stewart & Carter, 2006).

The ISAK accreditation scheme is based on the principles of certification, measurement experience and continuous practice, all of which serve to minimise measurement error. It recognises individuals of differing experience in a four-level hierarchy. A key element is the objective maintenance of quality assurance by requiring that individuals at all levels have to meet initial technical error of measurement (TEM) criteria in an end-of-course practical examination followed by the meeting of further TEM criteria on the measurement of 20 subjects to indicate satisfactory repeatability of measures.

The TEM is the approach ISAK has selected to quantify error in performing and repeating anthropometric measurements. The absolute TEM is calculated as follows:

$$\text{TEM} = \sqrt{\frac{\Sigma d^2}{2n}}$$

where Σd^2 is the sum of squared differences between measurements and n is the number of participants measured. The absolute TEM is multiplied by 100 and divided by the 'variable average value' (overall mean of the means between measurements of each participant for the same site) to provide the relative TEM (%TEM) for each site of measurement (Perini, de Oliveira, Ornellas & de Oliveira, 2005). The target inter- and intra-tester %TEMs required for different levels of ISAK accreditation are provided in Table 10.1. These targets are minimum requirements and in practice it is common to see accomplished ISAK practitioners with TEM scores well below these – for instance below 3 per cent and 2 per cent for inter- and intra-tester skinfolds, respectively.

Inter-tester candidate scores are analysed relative to a current qualified Level 3 or 4 (Level 4 in the case of Level 3 candidates).

TABLE 10.1 Target inter- and intra-tester %TEMs

Level	Assessment	Skinfolds	Other measurements
1	Inter-tester (exam)	12.5%	2.5%
	Intra-tester (exam)	10.0%	2.0%
	Intra-tester (post-exam)	7.5%	1.5%
2–4	Inter-tester (exam)	5.0%	1.0%
	Intra-tester (exam)	7.5%	1.5%
	Intra-tester (post-exam)	5.0%	1.0%

Each of the four levels of accreditation serves a different purpose, explained in more detail in the following subsections. Each level requires the ability to demonstrate 'landmarking', in which measurement sites are identified on the body, equipment manipulation, and knowledge of a profile of measurements, which is reduced, or 'restricted' at Level 1, and full (see Section 10.8) for subsequent levels.

Level 1 Anthropometrist (Technician – restricted profile)

Level 1 accreditation is designed for the majority of ISAK-accredited anthropometrists who have little ongoing requirement for more than the measurement of stature, body mass and skinfolds. Selected girths and two bone breadths are included to enable the monitoring of health and growth variables and calculation of the somatotype, which ISAK sees as valuable tools for the comparison of body size, shape and composition. A person who successfully completes Level 1 is able to demonstrate a basic understanding of the theory of anthropometric applications and can demonstrate adequate and competence in the two base measures, eight skinfolds, five girths and two breadth measurements covered by the restricted profile (Appendix 10.1). The Level 1 anthropometrist qualification equips individuals to perform these primary measures, which are routinely used with clinical groups and athletes.

Accreditation is achieved through the successful completion of a practical examination at the end of the Level 1 course and the post-course (within six months) completion of the restricted profile on 20 individuals, where each individual is landmarked and duplicate or triplicate measures taken. Certification expires four years and six months from the date of the practical examination, following which re-accreditation may be achieved through a further practical examination and the completion of the restricted profile on 20 individuals. Re-accreditation is also valid for a period of four years six months from the date of the practical examination.

Level 2 Anthropometrist (Technician – full profile)

Level 2 accreditation is designed for anthropometrists who wish to offer their subjects a more comprehensive range of 42 measurements. A Level 2 anthropometrist has a broad understanding of the theory of anthropometry and its interpretation, and can demonstrate adequate precision in the four base measures, eight skinfolds, nine segment lengths, 13 girths and eight breadths included in the full profile (Appendix 10.2, Section 10.8). The Level 2 anthropometrist qualification is the minimum requirement for technicians measuring for major anthropometric surveys endorsed by ISAK.

Level 2 candidates must have been accredited at Level 1 for a minimum of six months (although this may be a shorter time if they hold other appropriate professional qualifications). Level 2 accreditation is achieved through the successful completion of a practical examination and post-course completion of the full profile on 20 individuals. As with the Level 1 qualification, certification expires four years and six months from the date of the practical examination, following which the anthropometrist may repeat the assessment processes in order to extend the accreditation a further four years.

Level 3 Anthropometrist (Instructor)

The Level 3 course is designed for those anthropometrists wishing to engage in the training and accreditation of Levels 1 and 2 anthropometrists. Its purpose is to increase the availability of training courses so that ISAK training may be offered to greater numbers of candidates worldwide. A Level 3 candidate can demonstrate adequate precision in the 42 anthropometric dimensions of the full profile and has sufficient theoretical and practical knowledge of anthropometry to be able to instruct and accredit Level 1 and 2 anthropometrists. In addition to the anthropometric content, the Level 3 course covers pedagogy, statistics and working with 'special' populations (see Section 10.4). Learning how to teach, demonstrate, fault correct, and provide guided learning in small groups is fundamental to being effective in an instructor's role. The other key skill set beyond that expected at lower levels concerns the administration of an ISAK course, the process for which is necessarily well structured, and summarised in Figure 10.2.

While the core teaching material is established in the syllabus for each level, many courses are for research practitioners and as such may be integrated with other body composition measurement skills. Level 3 candidates must be a member of ISAK and meet the following prerequisites:

- Bachelor's degree or equivalent in human movement science, nutrition, sports medicine, medicine, functional anatomy or similar
- Completion of an ISAK Level 2 course
- Significant experience in anthropometry, equivalent to 100 full profiles (or judged as equivalent by a Level 4 anthropometrist).

In addition to a practical examination and completion of the full profile on 20 individuals, assessment at Level 3 includes a two to three hour written theory examination. Certification expires four years and six months from the date of the

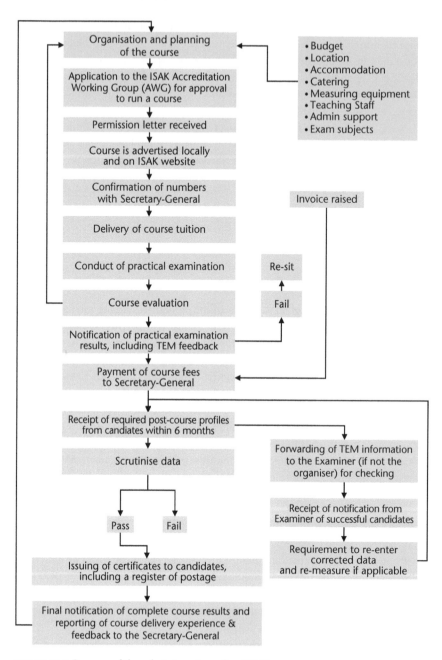

FIGURE 10.2 Process of the administration of an ISAK course.

practical examination or upon expiry of ISAK membership, whichever is the lesser period. Re-accreditation requires passing a practical examination, the successful completion of repeat measures of the full profile on 20 individuals, and evidence of ongoing involvement in the teaching and examining of ISAK courses. Re-accreditation is valid for four years from the date of completion of all re-accreditation requirements or, again, until the expiry of ISAK membership.

Level 4 Anthropometrist (criterion anthropometrist)

Level 4 is the most senior level, recognising many years of experience in taking ISAK-approved measurements, a high level of theoretical knowledge, involvement in the teaching/examining of ISAK workshops or courses, involvement in large anthropometric projects and a significant publication record in anthropometry. It is reserved for a relatively small group of anthropometrists and carries with it the responsibility to train and examine Level 3 anthropometrists, as well as the right to train and examine the other two levels.

Level 4 accreditation expires after a period of four years or upon expiry of ISAK membership, whichever date is the earlier. In order to gain re-accreditation to teach and examine ISAK accreditation courses, a criterion anthropometrist must request an extension for a further four years and provide evidence that s/he continues to meet criteria, including evidence of ongoing involvement in the teaching and examining of ISAK courses (in particular the running of, or involvement in, at least two Level 3 courses in the previous four years). Re-accreditation is valid for four years from the date of completion of all re-accreditation requirements, or until the expiry of ISAK membership.

Beyond this hierarchy, the wider membership has a forum for sharing knowledge, ideas, research, techniques and new developments in equipment and software. This is made much easier via the ISAK website (www.isakonline.com), internet forums, publications and conferences. While ISAK's practitioners in over 50 countries will be the first to admit that this method is not the only way of conducting anthropometric measurement, the 'ISAK method' quality assures data, standardises protocols and enables individuals from different parts of the world to collaborate. As science becomes more rigorous, such standardisation is likely to be adopted more widely among other body composition methods.

10.6 Best practice example: BASES

Founded in 1984, the British Association of Sport and Exercise Sciences (BASES; formerly BASS) is the professional body for sport and exercise sciences in the UK. The Association defines sport and exercise science as 'the application of scientific principles to the promotion, maintenance and enhancement of sport and exercise related behaviours', and has the following objectives:

- the promotion of research in sport and exercise sciences
- the encouragement of evidence-based practice in sport and exercise sciences
- the distribution of knowledge in sport and exercise sciences
- the development and maintenance of high professional standards for those involved in sport and exercise sciences
- the representation of the interests of sport and exercise sciences nationally and internationally.

(BASES, 2011a)

In order to promote evidence-based practice and high professional skills and standards, BASES provides a professional accreditation scheme, which is generally completed through a supervised experience process, although some candidates may have accrued sufficient professional experience to enable them to apply directly for accreditation. Body composition analysis is one field in which candidates may choose to specialise. Candidates must demonstrate competency in the following areas relevant to their domain of expertise:

- Scientific knowledge
- Technical skills
- Application of knowledge and skills
- Understanding and use of research
- Self-evaluation and professional development
- Communication
- Problem solving and impact
- Management of self, others and practice
- Understanding of the delivery environment
- Professional relationships and behaviours.

(BASES, 2011b)

There are many ways in which evidence may be given to demonstrate competency in the required areas. For example, scientific knowledge may be demonstrated by providing evidence of recognised qualifications such as degree certificates. The application of knowledge and skills may be demonstrated through case studies and reflective accounts. Other forms of evidence may include, but are not limited to, conference presentations, training course attendance and client testimonials.

In addition to the identified requirements, candidates must be familiar with ethical guidelines and are bound by the provisions of the code of conduct. The BASES code of conduct highlights principles of professionalism, integrity and safety, and incorporates aspects such as ethical clearance, informed consent and confidentiality, data protection, competence and personal conduct. Violations of the code can result in sanctions, including withdrawal of accreditation. The full code of conduct can be viewed online: www.bases.org.uk/Publications-Documents-and-Policies.

Candidates on Supervised Experience require a supervisor or team of supervisors who have been BASES accredited for a minimum of three years or can demonstrate relevant experience, and have completed a BASES Supervisor workshop. The supervised experience process may take between two and six years to complete. Candidates must attend a number of BASES workshops and complete 500 hours of logged supervised practice. An Accreditation Competency Profile must be completed, demonstrating how competencies have been achieved and detailing at least one case study, along with evidence of other relevant qualifications such as degree certificates. Applicants must also submit references from a mentor and two clients. All applications for Accreditation are judged by the Accreditation Committee. Accreditation is awarded for five years, after which individuals may apply for re-accreditation. Further information pertaining to the BASES accreditation scheme, along with contact details, may be found on the BASES website (www.bases.org.uk).

10.7 Partnerships and future directions

Scientific enquiry has always enabled individuals from different places to work together on a common idea. This phenomenon prevails in all disciplines, and in body composition the variety of applications and 'host disciplines' is arguably as great as anywhere. However, it is important to recognise that ours is a relatively young discipline, which as yet lacks the legal and financial frameworks, and governance structures of professional organisations of more mature disciplines. We must recognise that the evolution of any professional organisation starts with interested individuals, be it the International Working Group on Kinanthropometry in 1978, which was replaced by ISAK in 1986, or the more recent International Society for Body Composition Research (ISBCR), which began in 2006. While BASES and ISAK are both training organisations that provide qualifications as well as being professional interest groups, ISBCR embraces areas that facilitate the path to maturity of body composition as a scientific discipline. Under its strategy, it hosts conferences for a range of professional groups, publishes an international journal, and seeks to standardise aspects of methodology. This makes perfect sense, given that of the score or so methods available to quantify body composition, an active practitioner could not be expected to join one organisation for each method. The ISBCR seeks to cross-validate new methods, and participate in large-scale trials, for which a common methodology is an essential prerequisite. This, in turn, will lead to normative values which stand a greater chance of adoption in participant countries. In addition, there is a need to seek partnerships with commercial organisations in order to encourage new technological developments. It is clear that in a competitive market, commercial confidentiality can mean that algorithms for calculating body composition are not in the public domain. However, in order to be of use to scientists, such methods need to be subjected to rigorous validation which is made more likely with larger, multi-centre investigations.

There are likely to be other developments relating to convergence of technologies, and the integration of data into multi-component models. While the economic aspects of future research remain uncertain, two things are well established. First, the cost of technology is falling. Second, our capacity to communicate and share data in a virtual environment is increasing. Both these factors suggest a healthy future for body composition research where these enabling technologies will catalyse developments and make our discipline vibrant, exciting and successful.

10.8 Sample forms

This section contains the following appendices:

Appendix 10.1: ISAK restricted profile (2011 protocol).

ANTHROPOMETRIC PROFORMA

Appendix 10.2: ISAK full profile (2011 protocol).

ANTHROPOMETRIC PROFORMA

Subject Name (first, last) _____   Subject ID# ☐☐☐

Country _____   Ethnicity _____   Sex _____   Sport _____

	Day	Month	Year	Time	
Date of Measurement	☐☐	☐☐	☐☐	☐☐	Measurer ☐
	Day	Month	Year		
Date of Birth	☐☐	☐☐	☐☐		Recorder ☐

		First measure	Second measure	Third measure	MEAN/MEDIAN
1	Body mass				
2	Stretch stature				
3	Sitting Height				
4	Arm Span				
5	Triceps sf				
6	Subscapular sf				
7	Biceps sf				
8	Iliac Crest sf				
9	Supraspinale sf				
10	Abdominal sf				
11	Front Thigh sf				
12	Medial Calf sf				
13	Head girth				
14	Neck girth				
15	Arm girth relaxed				
16	Arm girth flexed and tensed				
17	Forearm girth (max. relaxed)				
18	Wrist girth (distal styloid)				
19	Chest girth (mesosternale)				
20	Waist girth (min.)				
21	Gluteal girth (max.)				
22	Thigh girth (1 cm dist. glut. line)				
23	Thigh girth (mid tro-tib lat)				
24	Calf girth (max.)				
25	Ankle girth (min.)				
26	Acromiale-radiale				
27	Radiale-stylion				
28	Midstylion-dactylion				
29	Iliospinale ht				
30	Trochanterion ht				
31	Trochanterion-tibiale laterale				
32	Tibiale laterale ht				
33	Tibiale mediale-sphyrion tibiale				
34	Biacromial breadth				
35	A-P Abdominal depth				
36	Billiocristal breadth				
37	Foot length (ak-pt)				
38	Transverse chest breadth				
39	A-P Chest depth				
40	Humerus breadth (biepicondylar)				
41	Styloid breadth (biepicondylar)				
42	Femur breadth (biepicondylar)				

Appendix 10.3: Sample consent form.

Ethics Committee   reference number: **/****/*****

(Form to be on headed paper)

Centre Number: Study Number:
Patient Identification Number for this trial:

CONSENT FORM

Title of Project:

Name of Researcher:

Please initial box

1.	I confirm that I have read and understand the information sheet dated .... (version ....) for the above study. I have had the opportunity to consider the information, ask questions and have had these answered satisfactorily.	
2.	I understand that my participation is voluntary and that I am free to withdraw at any time, without giving any reason, without my medical care or legal rights being affected.	
3.	I understand that relevant sections of any of my medical notes and data collected during the study, may be looked at by responsible individuals from the *************** University from regulatory authorities or from the NHS Trust, where it is relevant to my taking part in this research. I give permission for these individuals to have access to my records.	
4.	I agree to my GP being informed of my participation in the study.	
5.	I agree that in the event of my withdrawal from the study, outcome data from my participation can be used.	
6	I understand that no images which may identify me can be used in any presentation or publication without my prior agreement	
7.	I agree to take part in the above study	

I agree to take part in the above study

_____   _____   _____

Name of Participant   Signature   Date

_____   _____   _____

Name of Person taking consent   Signature   Date
(if different from researcher)

When completed, 1 for patient; 1 for researcher site file; 1 (original) to be kept in medical notes

Appendix 10.4: Basic risk assessment form (reproduced with permission from the Safety Adviser's Office, University of Liverpool, Liverpool, UK).

THE UNIVERSITY OF LIVERPOOL
RISK ASSESSMENT

Department	Location

Description of project/task

Person(s) involved and status

Main hazards of the work/project *(Consider: people who can be affected, equipment used, materials handled and environment hazards)*	Controls required *(Consider: appropriate physical, procedural and behavioural controls).*

Level of Supervision (circle)	A = Work may not be started without direct supervision B = Work may not start without the supervisor's advice or approval C = No specific extra supervision requirements

Other relevant specific assessments (List)

Date for review of assessment (maximum period of 5 years)
Hazards identified and precautions specified are appropriate for the task
Head of Department/DSC/Academic supervisor Signature.. Date...................

Acknowledgement by person(s) involved..

A copy of this assessment should be sent to the Departmental Safety Coordinator. The Management of Health and Safety at Work Regulations require that a risk assessment is carried out before work starts. For guidance on risk assessment see Safety Circular SC42/3.

ALWAYS REVIEW THE ASSESSMENT IF CIRCUMSTANCES CHANGE.
DON'T WAIT FOR THE FORMAL REVIEW.

References

BASES (2011a). *The British Association of Sport and Exercise Sciences: Strategy 2011–2014.* www.bases.org.uk/write/documents/BASESstrategicplan2011-2014for%20web.pdf [accessed June 2011].

BASES (2011b). *Accreditation Competency Profile.* www.bases.org.uk/Accreditation/ Accreditation [accessed December 2011].

Department of Health (2000). *Ionising Radiation (Medical Exposure) Regulations.* Statutory Instrument 2000 Number 1059. London: The Stationery Office. [Also available online at www.dh.gov.uk/en/Publicationsandstatistics/Publications/PublicationsPolicyAnd Guidance/DH_4007957].

HSE (2011). Five steps to risk assessment. *Leaflet INDG163 (rev3).* Suffolk: HSE Books. [Also available online at www.hse.gov.uk/risk/fivesteps.htm].

ISCS (International Society for Clinical Densitometry). (2007). *ISCD 2007 Official Positions and Pediatric Official Positions.* Middletown, CT: ISCD.

Madsen, O.R., Lorentzen, J.S., Lauridsen, U.B., Egsmose, C. and Sorensen, O.H. (2000). Effects of silicone breast prostheses on the assessment of body composition. *Clinical Physiology, 20,* 279–282.

Marfell-Jones, M., Olds, T., Stewart, A. and Carter, J.E.L. (2006). *International Anthropometry Accreditation Scheme Handbook.* Potchefstroom: ISAK.

National Commission for the Protection of Human Subjects of Biomedical and Behavioral Research (1979). *The Belmont Report: Ethical Principles and Guidelines for the Protection of Human Subjects of Research.* http://ohsr.od.nih.gov/guidelines/belmont.html [accessed June 2011].

NIH (National Institutes of Health). (2004). *Guidelines for the Conduct of Research Involving Human Subjects.* http://ohsr.od.nih.gov/guidelines/GrayBooklet82404.pdf [accessed June 2011].

Perini, T.A., de Oliveira, G.L., Ornellas, J.S. and de Oliveira, F.P. (2005). Technical error of measurement in anthropometry. *Revista Brasileira de Medicina do Esporte, 11,* 86–90.

Ryan, P.J. (2003). Setting up a bone density service. *Osteoporosis Review, 11,* 1–5.

INDEX